THE
Cancer Epidemic:
SHADOW OF THE
CONQUEST OF NATURE

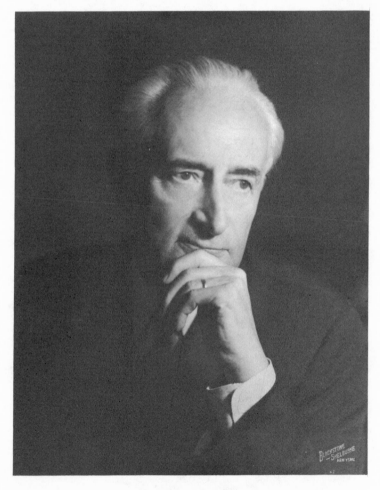

Gotthard Booth

THE
Cancer Epidemic:
SHADOW OF THE CONQUEST OF NATURE

By
GOTTHARD BOOTH

The Edwin Mellen Press
New York and Toronto

Library of Congress Catalogue Card Number   A 597362
ISBN 0-88946-625-4

Typesetting and design services by the Open Studio, Ltd., Rhinebeck & Barrytown, N.Y.

The Edwin Mellen Press
Suite 918
225 West 34th Street
New York, New York 10001

Editors' Note

When Dr. Booth died in November 1975, his archives were moved to Wilfrid Laurier University and its affiliated college, Waterloo Lutheran Seminary, where Dr. Booth had directed annual seminars on Religion and Health since 1965.

In 1977 The Gotthard Booth Society for Holistic Health was established in order to promote studies and activities related to Dr. Booth's legacy. This Society and the New York Psychosomatic Cancer Study Group (Dr. Charles Weinstock) have supported the publication of the present volume. Dr. M. Darrol Bryant saw the manuscript through to publication.

In editing this volume, both the original 1963 manuscript and the larger 1974 manuscript were consulted. In addition, a 1975 revision (some of it handwritten by the author) was followed. The references, not complete in any extant manuscript, were completed by checking the author's published and unpublished papers as well as the files and the library he left behind. In this way, also, the texts of the appendix and some notes missing from the manuscripts were found.

Aarne Siirala
Professor of Religion
Wilfrid Laurier University

Tom Foster
Secretary
The Gotthard Booth Society for Holistic Health
Waterloo, Ontario, Canada

Foreword

Pronouncements concerning the relationship between mind and body have appeared in different settings scattered throughout the literature of the world, from ancient times to the present day. The numerous ideas and theories pertaining to the "psyche" and the "soma" have usually implied that they are separate entities with a certain amount of interaction between them, rather than considering them as different aspects or components of a single biological unity.

At present, just as modern atomic and subatomic research in physics is rapidly removing the conceptual boundaries which were once thought to distinguish energy and matter, physiological and psychological researches are well on the way to erase the, once assumed, frontier between mind and body concepts. Modern experimental and clinical researches are progressively filling in the details of the manner in which emotional states produce a wide variety of disturbances of function, and under certain conditions produce such organic responses which are irreversible, leading to the formation of pathological lesions in the bodily structure.

Since there are numerous individual differences in the expression of disease, in the emotional organization, and in behavior patterns involving the three categories of behavior, viz: biochemical (metabolic), locomotor (neuro-muscular), and psychological (thought, emotion, etc.), it seems rather obvious that the chain of events occurs in, or is a part of, a special personality response. The soma and the psyche have evolved together as a unit, as a constellation, in the same individual. The behavior of the organism as a unit with its structure, adaptations, and its disorders is apparently the result of the slow development of a series of discharging functions into this unit that begins at conception and continues through the years. Therefore, it would seem that somatobiological, psychobiological, and sociobiological forces are all actively integrated together in the manifestations of health and disease.

The integrations of tissue, temperament, and personality dynamics out of which, under special circumstances, there emerge characteristic reactions, including somatopathological and psychopathological conditions, deserve and invite further investigation.

In this excellent account of careful investigation and scholarly reporting, the author presents his studies of persons who have developed the serious disease: cancer. He has brought together a noteworthy number of observations and an experimental approach, the results of which are given in categories of Rorschach responses.

At the present time, the Rorschach technique, when administered by an expert, such as the author of this research, is considered in most psychiatric and psychologic clinics to be a remarkably accurate means of gaining information about a patient's personality in terms of intellectual function, emotional control, present content, mental conflicts, creative imagination, and fundamental instinctive drives. It is an accepted procedure for both routine and research work. It is a projective test in which each patient gives his own interpretation of otherwise meaningless, but standardized, figures. Because these figures are forms of no apparent significance, the subject has no objective way of controlling his reactions to the test material. Therefore, the interpretation of each figure must derive from the subject himself; thus, the manner in which the material stimulates or releases associative processes can serve, when scored, as a basis for individual personality evaluation.

From these studies and from the known aspects of the cancer situation the author suggests that cancer is an expression of the personality type and that the cancer patient is dominated by anal components. In this the personality differs from that in the tuberculosis situation. It appears conclusive that the specific dynamisms manifest themselves also through the life histories of the two groups, thus perhaps indicating the predisposition or habitus that becomes traumatized by the disease. Modern medical science is piling up evidence of the special uniqueness of the individual, but by sorting out and classifying reactions one finds some common denominators that allow the grouping of different patterns of both physiological functions and psychological behavior.

The wide publicity given to statistical surveys of cigarette and other tobacco habits in terms of an etiological factor in lung cancer has relegated to the background many other basic observations on other possible components, particularly in the sphere of the personality and emotional constellations. The author has given many excellent suggestions and implications which merit further investigation, and research-minded physicians who can deal with both personality function and the functions of organ systems of the body have a unique opportunity of observing human behavior living out the biographical events with their psychological and social implications.

The time has passed in the history and progress of medicine when the belief was practically universal that any context that can be understood in terms of an organic process or disease has no psychological determinants, components, implications, or influence.

The report is rich in new ideas, and, allowing for some generalizations and even some speculations, there is a wealth of informative material to be considered in practical applications, not only in the field of psychopathology but also in general medicine.

Nolan D. C. Lewis, M.D.

Acknowledgements

The research underlying the present monograph was sponsored by the Department of Psychiatry, College of Physicians and Surgeons, of Columbia University, at that time under the leadership of Nolan D.C. Lewis, M.D., Director of the New York Psychiatric Institute. After his retirement Dr. Lewis maintained his interest in the development of my work, and I am particularly grateful for his preceding introduction to the final publication.

Lenore Korkes, Ph.D., administered the Rorschach tests to the first 15 lung cancer patients and to the 82 tuberculosis patients who were the subjects of her doctoral thesis on the prognosis of pulmonary tuberculosis (1955). Her careful records made the present study possible. The cooperating agencies included the New York Tuberculosis and Health Association, the Department of Health of the City of New York, the New York State Division of Vocational Rehabilitation and the following hospitals in the City of New York: Bellevue, Delafield, Memorial, Seton and the Washington Heights Chest Clinic.

Miriam Shrifte, Ph.D., contributed 50 additional Rorschach records of cancer patients when it became apparent that the original comparative study of cancer and tuberculosis of the lungs had relevance to the cancer problem in general. Of these patients, 49 had cancer of organs other than the lungs. All of them had been studied for the purpose of establishing psychological variables in host resistance to cancer (1962). Dr. Shrifte's work was done with the cooperation of the Surgical Division of Bellevue Hospital in Hew York. This generous support of my investigation into the personality structure of cancer was uniquely in contrast to the lack of response from other authors who had published reports on various aspects of the Rorschach responses of cancer patients.

Other contributors of Rorschach records of unselected cancer patients were: E. Kuntz-Evers, M.D., Städtisches Krankenhaus Ost in Lübeck, Germany; Molly Harrower, Ph.D., and John Goss, M.D., in New York, N.Y.

My wife, Edith E. Booth, drew the pictures of some of the Rorschach percepts which differentiate between the two clinical groups. These illustrations proved very helpful in conveying essential points to professional audiences and readers of preliminary articles (Booth, 1964b, 1965).

My daughter, Beatrice Hudson, contributed a great deal to the manuscript by editing and typing its various stages.

The initial phase of the study was aided financially by the late Mrs. Dorothy Tillmann in memory of her husband Georg. It was her intuition, back in 1942, that scientific research could prove the critical role of psychological and religious factors in the pathogenesis of cancer. Unfortunately she died before Dean Willard C. Rapleye Jr. had accepted her project and bequest on behalf of Columbia University.

The following chapters are partly based on previous publications: "Voice of the Body" in *The Voice of Illness* by Aarne Siirala, (Fortress Press, Philadelphia, 1964); "Cancer and Humanism" in *Psychosomatic Aspects of Neoplastic Disease,* Editors: D.M. Kissen and L.L. LeShan, Lippincott, Philadelphia, 1964) and articles in the following journals: *Ztschr. f. Psychosomatische Medizin, Am. J. Psyshanal., J. Am. Med. Assoc., Pastoral Psychology, Ann. N.Y. Acad. Sci.,* and *J. Am. Acad. of Psychoanalysis.*

The original manuscript was finished in 1963 and read by Dr. Nolan D.C. Lewis and Dr. Lawrence Kolb. At the time publishers considered the psychobiological approach to the cancer problem too controversial to accept it. Since then ten years passed and I had opportunity for developing the material and for presenting various parts of it to professional groups in America and in Europe.

I wish to thank the many specialists who read the parts of the manuscript which called for their expertise: Dr. Molly Harrower and Miriam Shrifte (Rorschach), Dr. Lawrence LeShan (Psychology of Cancer), Dr. René Dubos (Biology), Joseph Campbell (Mythology), Dr. Margaret Mead and Dr. Hortense Powdermaker (Anthropology) and Dr. Aarne Siirala (Theology). I paid close attention to their opinions and trust that their cooperation made the manuscript a responsible contribution to the cancer problem.

Gotthard Booth, 1974

Contents

◆

List of Plates, Tables and Figures

"The whole understanding of the world consists in the analysis of process in terms of the identities and diversities of the individuals involved. The peculiarities of the individuals are reflected in the peculiarities of the common process which is their interconnection. We can start our investigation from either end; namely, we can characterize the process and then consider the characterization of the individuals; or we can characterize the individuals and conceive them as formative of the relevant process. In truth, the distinction is only one of emphasis."

Alfred North Whitehead
Modes of Thought

Introduction

Clinical Premises
and Scope of the Present Investigation

Since the middle of the 19th century, the number of deaths from cancer among the Caucasian populations of Europe, Australia, and New Zealand has been rising at the same rate at which tuberculosis mortality has been declining.

This phenomenon was first observed by Sir Thomas Coglan in 1902, but it did not become part of the medical thinking of the period. Twenty years later (1924/1925) Thomas Cherry rediscovered the phenomenon and gave it a precise formulation: *The sum of tuberculosis and cancer deaths amounts to 20 percent of the total mortality of the adult population.* This ratio was not affected either by the great socio-economic changes during the seven decades surveyed by Cherry or by the many differences of climate under which the 11 sample populations had been living.

The findings certainly were intriguing; but, again, they did not become part of the medical concepts of the two diseases. Thirty-five years later (1960), Joseph Berkson examined American statistics and found that the spectacular rise of lung cancer since 1930 had been compensated by the equivalent decline in tuberculosis deaths. In 1963, J.T. Haybittle confirmed Cherry's work on the basis of the British mortality statistics since Cherry's original publication.

The two diseases are histologically and clinically so dissimilar, however, that investigators in somatic medicine, with its cytological bias, made no attempt to look into the nature of the link between them. To the best of my knowledge, nobody proposed what seems to me the most plausible explanation: *Tuberculosis and cancer are two alternate liabilities of a genotype that occurs in 20 percent of Caucasian populations* (Booth, 1967b, 1969b).

This hypothesis has important practical implications:

1. The current cancer epidemic is approaching a definite ceiling.
2. Carcinogenic agents do not threaten everybody, but only 20 percent of the adult population.
3. There is, at least theoretically, the possibility of diagnosing tuberculosis-prone and cancer-prone individuals.

The concept of a common genetic predisposition of cancer and tuberculosis victims is supported by studies of the incidence of cancer in 300 families observed by A.S. Warthin between 1895 and 1925, a period when tuberculosis was still endemic. Warthin noted that tuberculosis was the disease most frequently occurring in cancer families, particularly in the case of cancer patients who had no cases of cancer in their ancestry.

Numerous publications have established the fact that lung cancer is frequently preceded by tuberculosis, but they have assumed a cause-effect relationship. More recently, however, evidence has been presented (Clifton and Irani, 1970) that in 82.54 percent of 292 tuberculosis patients the neoplasia originated in organs *other* than the lungs and larynx, suggesting a coincidence of cancer and tuberculosis liability.

The experimental cancer research of Jonas Salk (1969) and of D.W. Weiss (1969) led to evidence that animals who have immunological defenses against tuberculosis are also protected against cancer implants. From the shared immunological behavior of tuberculosis and cancer, the conclusion may be drawn that both diseases belong to a genetic group set apart from the rest of the population by instability of defenses against the mycobacterium tuberculosis and the many carcinogenic agents.[1] As far as *cancer* is concerned, R. Doll pointed out in a recent survey (1965) that even powerful carcinogenic agents do not necessarily cause neoplasia. He gave the striking example of the 2,500 residents of Hiroshima and Nagasaki who survived the explosion of the atomic bombs within 1,100 meters of the hypocenter. Fewer than 2 percent developed leukemia, a figure high enough to indicate the leukemogenic effect of radiation, but also low enough to establish the importance of other factors, among them the genetic disease predisposition. For tuberculosis, this was demonstrated by the Lübeck catastrophe of 1926 (Dubos, 1959). In this instance, 249 babies were vaccinated inadvertently with enormous numbers of virulent bacilli. Whereas 35 percent died from acute tuberculosis, 65 percent survived and were found to be free of the disease 12 years later.

No cancerogenic agent, apparently, leads invariably to neoplasia in human beings. Furthermore, as documented by Everson and Cole (1966), even without medical intervention, in some instances cancer does not run a fatal course but may remain stationary or even disappear.

Sir David Smithers, a leading English oncologist, asserted (1964) that the complexity of neoplasia cannot be understood if one treats the problem as localized in the cells that undergo neoplastic changes. He came to the following conclusion:

> "What we need most at the present is to develop an autonomous science of organismal organization, the social science of the human body...willing to recognize that whole functioning organisms are its proper concern. Overgrowth and dedifferentiation are effects of disorganization—*repercussions, not driving forces.* Cancer is no more a disease of cells than a traffic jam is a disease of cars. A lifetime of study of the internal combustion engine would not help anyone to understand our traffic problems. A traffic jam is due to a failure of normal relationships between driven cars and their environment."

Smithers based his organismic concept of cancer on somato-biological considerations. The results of my own psycho-biological research confirm the hypothesis that *cancer can be understood as localized repercussion of a traumatic encounter between a specific type of organism—the cancer-prone individual—and specific environmental conditions.*

Smither's concept added a new dimension to the study of neoplastic disease: the *ethological* clarification of cancer as specific biological behavior released by specific elements of the environment. Ethological studies of animals (Tinbergen, 1955) have demonstrated that only a few schematic elements of their natural environment release the behavior by which they survive. That even in homo sapiens such primitive schemata are effective, Konrad Lorenz has demonstrated.

At the time of Smither's attack on "cytologism" in cancer research, I had completed the experimental part of an investigation of the subject-environment relationships of cancer patients. Hermann Rorschach's psychodiagnostic method had been chosen because it confronts every subject with the same ten standard objects: pictures of nonrepresentational inkblots which, on an unconscious level, suggest 10 different existential situations. The percepts of the individual subjects necessarily reflect both personality and environment as a unit, formed by the subjective image and the objective elements of the inkblot that elicited the image.

The observation of specific perceptual tendencies prevailing in all cancer patients made it possible to isolate cancer-related responses from among the great number of responses which confirm that, in many other respects, cancer patients are very unlike each other. Evidently, the disease-specific percepts result from an unconscious selective scanning process analogous to the instinctual capacity of animals to respond to the grotesque dummies of ethologists as if they were natural objects. The findings were further clarified by comparing the group of cancer patients with a group of tuberculosis patients.

The methodology and the results of my research were presented in 1960 at the first meeting of the International Psychosomatic Cancer Research Group, which had been organized by Drs. Lawrence LeShan (U.S.A), David Kissen (Scotland), and Joachim Baltrusch (West Germany). The favorable response to my contribution encouraged me to prepare a monograph giving a detailed account of work, so as to make control studies possible and to develop fully various implications of the perceptanalytical approach for specific clinical problems of oncology. I offered the manuscript to 10 reputable scientific publishers, with the backing of Nolan D.C. Lewis, who had originally provided the opportunity of studying cancer and tuberculosis patients (Booth, 1965). All the publishers ultimately rejected the manuscript, two of them expressing openly their regret that they had to follow the advice of their public relations executives. At that time the overwhelming majority of the medical profession and of the general public desperately believed that "the conquest of cancer" would be achieved by cytological research, being particularly encouraged by the statistical data on the association between cigarette smoking and lung cancer.

Since it seemed to me it would probably be a waste of time to try more publishing houses, I began to use the manuscript as source material for a number of articles and congress contributions. These appeared between 1963 and 1975 in the United States and in various European countries. Now there is evidence that the climate of opinion has become more favorable toward psychobiological cancer research, and that a revision of the monograph may find a publisher.

The first four chapters use the experimental data of the first manuscript. The last 14 years have provided opportunity for checking my method of Rorschach evaluation against many records shown to me by interested colleagues, and I have not come across any records contradicting my original findings that the cancer-prone and the tuberculosis-prone personalities can be differentiated from each other on the basis of objective perceptanalytical criteria. The psychological interpretation of the criteria has been clarified and should be easy to follow, even for readers unfamiliar with the Rorschach method.

The next chapters integrate the perspectives gained from the Rorschach analysis with the results of other pertinent studies. They try to convey an *anthropological concept of cancer* that goes beyond the individual encounter with the disease and that traces the origin of the epidemic to the historical changes in the relationship between man and nature (Chapters V and VI). These developments eventually led to the fatal role of the Industrial Revolution in creating a growing number of cancer-prone individuals (Chapter VII).

Chapter VIII deals with the psychobiological conditions that make specific body organs primary sites of the disease and discusses the complex interplay of biological and psychological factors in the link between lung cancer and cigarette smoking. The ninth chapter clarifies the psychobiological factors that can support the patient in his struggle against the disease and account for the enormous variety of outcomes: at one extreme, those who rapidly succumb in spite of early and expert therapy; at the other extreme, those who "spontaneously" recover after they have been given up by all medical experts.

Finally, in Chapter X the future of the cancer epidemic is considered in the light of the profound biological, cultural, and infantile roots of the neoplastic expression of life among the emotionally most vulnerable members of industrialized societies. Cytological medical science has amply demonstrated its limited effectiveness in preventing or curing cancer, but, because physical science has been designated an article of faith, frequently replacing any other religion, most people seem to hang on superstitiously to animistic slogans such as "war against cancer" and "destroying the invader." In recent years, however, a growing number of physicians (though still a minority) have become concerned with the psycho-social aspects of the disease. At the same time, new trends in the values of contemporary society assert themselves. They begin to counter-balance the influence of the ideology that in the last two centuries has favored the epidemic spread of the disease, which used to be rare.

Although the clues to the understanding of the cancer problem were found in the responses of tuberculosis and cancer patients to the Rorschach inkblots, readers not interested in this psychodiagnostic method may skip the first four chapters because the contents of Chapters V through X are documented by independent material. There are, however, several reasons why I consider the experimental part of this work too important to relegate to an appendix for the benefit of Rorschach specialists:[2]

1. The great value of Rorschach's psychodiagnostic experiment as applied to the study of somatic diseases should be appreciated more widely than is presently the case. Concrete demonstration of the use of the method in analyzing the dynamics of tuberculosis and cancer should encourage application of the method to other somatic diseases.

2. *The method for evaluating Rorschach imagery in organic diseases differs considerably from the method commonly used by clinical psychologists for evaluating psychiatric patients.* Physicians and psychologists cannot obtain comparable results unless they use the same perceptanalytical criteria. Even in evaluating psychiatric patients, the added dimensions of somatic dynamics definitely improve the value of Rorschach tests, as I know from ample experience with physically healthy subjects (Booth, 1960, 1963a, 1963b).

3. The Rorschach method provides more information than the evidence that a given patient belongs to a certain diagnostic category. Most individual records also contain specific *clues to the precise nature of the existential conflict that is relevant* in the particular case. The half-hour spent on administering the test is apt to save many hours otherwise spent on verbal probing.

The claims made for the unique value of the newly added dimensions of Rorschach analysis are well supported by the results of the present cancer study. In the course of the last 20 years, many experienced psychiatrists, clinical psychologists, and Rorschach experts have studied cancer patients without discovering the basic dynamics underlying the manifold forms of the disease. Their handicap has been the deep-seated Cartesian delusion of Western man: that the psyche is an immaterial individual entity that encounters the material reality of the external world.

This Cartesian prejudice has limited most psychological studies of somatic patients to observation of their subjective reactions to their objective physical disturbances. These disturbances are still widely considered to be caused by the impact of noxious physical agencies, unrelated to the personalities of the victims, on "normal" organs.

Medicine has only very slowly begun to revise its physicalistic concept of disease. Seventy years have gone by since Albert Einstein successfully revolutionized physics, the ideal model of scientific medicine, by *introducing the subject* into the study of material events. Although Einstein's theory affected only the impersonal field of physics and did not disturb the main body of that discipline, he at first encountered resistance from many colleagues. The resistance revealed Western man's anxious dependency on faith in the absolute nature of autonomous matter.

For medicine, the introduction of the subject constituted a far more serious threat. There were fewer scientific certainties concerning the course of somatic diseases, and their practical application involved awesome personal responsibilities. Thus, there were ample theoretical and practical reasons why the growing specialty of psychosomatic research stopped short of studying *the role of the subject in all forms of somatic disease.* Whenever the course of a somatic disease revealed the influence of psychological factors, the latter were treated as secondary complications of the primary physical pathology. In a materialistic culture, somatic data appeared more trustworthy. As Henri Ellenberger observed (1970): "Curing the sick is not enough; one must cure them with methods accepted by the community."

The first step toward the introduction of the subject into scientific medical research was made in 1946 by Viktor von Weizsäcker when he published *Der Gestaltkreis: Theorie der Einheit von Wahrnehmen und Bewegen* (The Gestalt Circle: Theory of the Unity of Perceiving and Moving). In this as yet untranslated book, he demonstrated, on the basis of exact neurophysiological experiments, that the subject is an integral part of biological dynamics. The theoretical analysis provided a concept of medicine that disposed of the old dichotomies of body and mind, of causalism and voluntarism, as effectively as modern physics had disposed of the dichotomy of mass and energy. The next step, from theory to clinical application, however, has proven most difficult to take.

For the scientist used to working in terms of quantifiable physical data, the very word "subject" had the connotation of "subjective." The concept of something existing only in the mind of the patient entailed an *a priori* prejudice that there could be no place for "the subject" in the world of objective data. Furthermore, there was the uncomfortable practical situation that responsible physicians were struggling with a rising flood of somatic information that made diagnostic and therapeutic decisions increasingly difficult. Under these circumstances, the practice of medicine threatened to become hopelessly unmanageable if the seemingly elusive "subject" should become an additional factor to be considered.

As a result of this state of modern medicine, there has been virtually no scientific interest in Rorschach's discovery that it is possible to *define subjects objectively on the basis of perceptanalytical data.* Somatic medicine has taken no interest in the fact that it is possible to define the psychodynamics of the subjects who develop specific diseases and to explain why they are adversely affected by specific physical and social factors that are not pathogenic for other types of subjects (Booth, 1946a, 1946b, 1948, 1964a, 1964b, 1964c, 1965). Even in the field of psychiatry, the majority of Rorschach's colleagues either ignored his method or allowed it to become the responsibility of clinical psychologists.

The development of Rorschach's intuitive discovery into a method for putting the study of the subject-environment relationship on a sound biological basis owes a great deal to the synchronous development of the new science of ethology. By one of the mysterious coincidences in the history of science (Booth, 1974c), Jacob von Uexküll published the final edition of *The Inner World and the Outer World of Animals* in the same year in which Rorschach published *Psychodiagnostics* — 1921. Two decades later it became apparent that perceptanalysts and ethologists dealt with the same aspect of life: *The biological structures of organisms are highly specific counterparts of equally specific elements of the environment.* The organism and its relevant objects fit each other like lock and key, exemplifying inuntold variations the worldwide intuitions of a pervasive harmony of nature. The rationale of the ethological concept of nature has made it possible to come to an understanding and acceptance of those manifestations that frighten modern materialists: disease and death (Booth, 1975).

This report emphasizes the idea that *the personal predisposition of the victim* is the one and only indispensable factor of the disease, determining the contingencies of life that trigger the development of neoplasia in a certain organ and at a certain time. The nature of some of those contingencies has been established as the result of the tremendous body of scientific knowledge accruing from the search for a specific cause of the disease. Many physical and chemical agents are statistically correlated with neoplasia; but neither do they prove carcinogenic for individuals equally exposed, nor is the timing of the disease explained by the physical facts.

The following chapters intend to clarify the role of molecular and biological conditions in the life history of cancer-prone individuals, who *all share the same core problem of loneliness.* They are born with the genetic handicap of an *abnormally strong need for affection* (Booth, 1969b), which obviously entails a high risk of infantile frustration. Many healthy mothers are constitutionally incapable of meeting abnormally strong affectional demands; others are handicapped, themselves, because of their own infantile experiences of inadequate mothering. Then there are the hazards of maternal illness, of economic adversity, and of constitutional incompatibility between infant and mother—Balint's "basic fault" (1968).

The experience of infantile affectional frustration causes these children to grow up without "basic trust" (Erikson, 1963), anxiously protecting themselves against having their feelings hurt. As adults, they become secretive and create their own social worlds where they feel in control of their emotional investments. Being generally strong, healthy personalities, they usually succeed in maintaining for many decades a way of life that satisfies their dominant needs.

The disease develops when these subjects realize that for some reason they have irretrievably lost the opportunity of keeping their idiosyncratic ways of life going. Such existential despair may come about as a result either of the devitalizing effect of aging or of traumatic changes in their external circumstances. Often both factors are in evidence.

At this point, the core problem of loneliness combined with secretiveness can become decisive for the prognosis of the disease. Even those closest to the patient are frequently unaware of what has driven him or her into the disease. Thus, often neither family nor friends nor physicians become alerted to the possibility of remedying the pathogenic situation (see Chapter X). This typical predicament has given rise to the widespread belief that cancer is a disease apt to strike anybody like lightning out of a blue sky. Consequently, fear of its surreptitious assault nowadays blights the life of the healthy and subjects cancer victims to misunderstandings that adversely affect their chances of being cured.

The following chapters provide scientific support and encouragement for the growing number of physicians and observant lay persons who are aware that psychological factors play a significant role in the results of somatic therapies. Even in the case of those who die of the disease, the humanistic approach can help patients to approach the end in a spirit of self-understanding, and in communication with understanding family members, friends, and physicians.

PART I

THE PERCEPTANALYTICAL DIFFERENTIATION OF CANCER AND TUBERCULOSIS

I

Somatic Disease and Perception

"Where all is fog, a blind man with a stick is
not entirely at a disadvantage."
— *I.W. Dunne*

A. *The Rationale of Rorschach's Psychodiagnostic Experiment*

In the course of the last 50 years, many psychiatrists have devoted
themselves to research in the field of somatic diseases. The pioneers of
psychosomatic medicine—Georg Groddeck, 1923; Nolan D.C. Lewis,
1924; Smith Ely Jelliffe and William Alanson White, 1935—understood all disease as a unitary process, as described by Lewis in his fore-
word to this book. The vast majority of the medical profession, however,
has continued to hold to the Cartesian concept of the dichotomy of
"soma" and "psyche." Although in theory there has been increasing
acknowledgment of the holistic character of life, in practice the distinction between "psychosomatic" and "purely somatic" diseases prevails.

Resistance against the unitary point of view is rooted in the
current identification of scientific medicine with a physico-chemical
interpretation of life. As Richard Doll remarked (1965): "That [psychic
factors] should have a direct effect on the development of cancer is not
an obviously attractive hypothesis."

The enormous prejudice in favor of purely somatological research is sustained by the fact that physical findings can be presented in terms of objective measurements. Psychological findings are always suspect of subjective bias because they are expressed in terms of personality traits abstracted from the interactions of patients with their undefined environments. Everybody knows from practical life experience that many people behave differently in the family, at work and at play, in their native environment and in confrontation with alien cultures, and, last but not least, in talking to different professionals (Jaffe and Slote, 1958).

Since not even monozygotic twins are completely alike in personality, and since environmental conditions can be equated only in respect of a few rough criteria, it is difficult to establish the relevance and objectivity of psychodynamic interpretations in the context of somatic pathology. Concepts derived from the dynamics of neuroses and psychoses do not necessarily apply to somatic processes that take place on a more deeply unconscious level — the unconscious that never was conscious (Sherrington, 1941).

The experimental psychodiagnostic method developed by Hermann Rorschach (1921) offers two obvious advantages in comparison with other methods of psychosomatic research:

1. The patients express their psychological reactions in forms that can be recorded objectively: their subjective percepts of 10 nonrepresentational inkblot pictures.
2. All patients are faced with exactly the same 10 environmental objects.

The basic principle of the method is illustrated by the example of a botanist and a zoologist walking together along the same trail through the woods. Inevitably, the one will notice more plants; the other, more animals. Faced with the inkblots, every individual is compelled to perceive them in terms of his own personality pattern. Rorschach's great discovery was the fact that the *content* of the percepts has only secondary diagnostic significance. Primary for the evaluation of the personality are purely formal criteria: the location of the percepts in the given inkblot and the roles of outline, color, shading, and kinesthesis in determining the percepts. In other words, the person looking at the inkblot is *consciously* preoccupied with finding similarities to concrete objects, but his *unconscious* dynamics limit him to certain formal patterns that are isomorphic with his personality structure. Illustrations will be found in Chapter II.

Recently, the physiological relationship between inkblot percepts and biological personality structure has been clarified by the ethological studies of animals. Specific instinctual behavior is elicited by very few of the many elements which, for the naive observer of the animal, constitute the appearance of the natural object (Tinbergen, 1955). Dummies embodying only the instinct-releasing features are as effective as the natural objects, although to us they may look grotesquely different. For instance, a male robin redbreast attacks furiously a bunch of red feathers placed in his breeding territory, but ignores a stuffed male bird whose breast has been painted grey. The dummy of a bird of prey scares chickens if it is moved head-first over the poultry yard, but produces no reaction if it is moved tail-first. Exaggerations of the normal stimulus make the dummy even more effective than the natural object. Brooding sea gulls, for instance, pay no attention to their own eggs if other eggs, too big to sit on, are placed next to the nesting site.

All instinctual behavior presupposes that the organism is in a biological state that makes the specific reaction purposeful: feeding presupposes hunger, copulating presupposes being in season. Sometimes the stimulus value of the same object changes abruptly: if the female spider is hungry at the time of copulation, the male becomes food immediately after the act.

The dummies of the ethologists owe their effectiveness to the peculiarity of instincts: in animals, the need for special *forms* of behavior prevails at the expense of the survival need of the individual. The end of purposive behavior is not the attainment of an object or a situation for itself, but the *performance of the consummatory action.* "Not the litter or the food is the animal striving toward, but the performance of maternal activities or eating" (Tinbergen, 1955). Human addictions illustrate the same phenomenon.

With the intuition of the true genius, Rorschach designed his 10 inkblot pictures in anticipation of what today has been learned from ethological research. The pictures fulfill for human beings the conditions that make the use of dummies a valuable method for analyzing animal behavior. Rorschach himself explained that he meant to create systematic variations of the aesthetic determinants he was interested in. Apparently he was not aware that he had created 10 *dummies of specific human situations.* He selected them from between 20 and 30 designs, on the empirical basis that they produced the most interesting responses.

Long after Rorschach's death, several researchers became aware of the secret of why the 10 inkblot pictures are uniquely effective, all working independently of each other and in different countries: Hector Ritey in Italy (1941), Ferencz Merei in Hungary (1953), F. Minkowska in France (1956), and I in this country.

Although the different authors define the demand character of the inkblot pictures somewhat differently, according to their psychological theories, in essence their conclusions agree. This will be discussed in Chapter III. For the purpose of the present chapter, the 10 plates may be characterized briefly as symbolizing the following situations: meeting the unknown; inescapable interpersonal confrontation; conventional interpersonal encounter; being without support in an anxiety-provoking situation; being alone in a banal situation; hetero-sexual encounter; interpersonal encounter without conventional social support; harmonious emotional situation; situation without opportunity for a satisfactory solution; and the future.

Each of the 10 pictures conveys, by means of nonrepresentational art, the unconscious experience of coping with a specific existential demand. At the same time, the nonrepresentational character of the inkblots creates *conscious anxiety* because the subject cannot find any forms fully representative of realistic objects. The resulting rational impasse leads to a state of tension that is analogous to the state of instinctual tension of an animal confronted with a dummy instead of the natural object of its need.

The animal finds relief from tension by responding to the instinct-releasers incorporated in the dummy. Man, "the rational animal," finds relief from his perceptual anxiety because the inkblots provide a practically infinite number of features that are *suggestive* of realistic objects.

Since none of the features add up to a *realistic representation* of any object, however, anxiety compels the subject to respond selectively to those features which offer an *approximate resemblance* to realistic objects. The latter, obviously, tend to be related to the manner in which the subject deals with the life situations suggested by the over-all design of the given inkblot picture. The creation of personally meaningful images from a few cues is a phenomenon analogous to the release of specific instinctual behavior in animals by dummies; in both cases, all contradictory visual data are ignored. (Chapters III and IV will provide illustrations of the process in human beings.)

The analogy between the release of animal instincts and the perception of the Rorschach pictures is not a mere figure of speech, but the manifestation of the biological functions which support the life of animals as well as that of the human species. The functional predominance of a specific biological function in a given individual expresses itself in the predominance of specific gestalt tendencies in his or her inkblot percepts. Unconsciously, biological dynamics structure the perceptual field. The personal life experiences of the subject only provide the specific contents of the Rorschach responses. (Examples are given in Chapter II and throughout Chapter III.) So far, clinical evidence has been published for the locomotor and the vasomotor functions (Booth, 1946a, 1946b), as well as for the pregenital and the genital functions (Booth, 1964b, 1964c, 1965).

The arousal of unconscious biological instincts explains the mysterious fascination (Tosquelles, 1945) which the inkblots exercise on nearly everybody.[3]

Several aspects of the Rorschach method are shared with the method of inducing hypnosis. In both, the ultimate purpose is mobilization of unconscious processes on the biological level of the subject. In both, the technique reduces the vigilance of the conscious mind:

1. Consciousness is narrowed in a general way by asking the subject to concentrate on a limited field of sensory awareness: the Rorschach plates, or the face and voice of the hypnotist.

2. In this general setting, the attention of the subject is directed toward phenomena that are directly accessible to his or her conscious experiences, and that actually have only an auxiliary function in respect of the mobilization of unconscious functions. The Rorschach subject is instructed to look for resemblances between the inkblots and real objects, a task that distracts him or her from any possible attention to the unconscious dynamics of his visual field. In hypnosis, the subject is instructed to concentrate on body experiences, such as breathing and temperature, distracting him or her from attention to the actual process of hypnosis.

For the purpose of studying the unconscious psychodynamics of somatic disease groups, the hypnotic element of the method is particularly important, because the patients are not aware that their frequently trivial percepts spell out basic self-revelations. Most somatic patients are disinclined to co-operate fully with psychological probing because our culture and modern medical practice rely on *physical* manipulation. Furthermore, a number of somatic patients realize their illness is related to personal situations that are either irreparable or too embarrassing to acknowledge.

In addition to these practical advantages, the Rorschach method has two unique advantages:

1. *The raw material for research is limited to the percepts that 10 standardized, nonrepresentational configurations elicit from the patients.*

The nonrepresentational character of the objects eliminates the influence of conventional and idiosyncratic associations that are bound to be evoked by the story-telling pictures of the Thematic Apperception Test and even more by strictly verbal tests. Furthermore, the productions of the subject are not influenced by individual variations of special talents for self-expression in verbal or in graphic form, such as are called upon by the T.A.T. and by various drawing tests, respectively. In the Rorschach performance, the subject does not create the basic material, and his perception of it is limited by constitutional factors. As a result, the gestalt tendencies in the different clinical groups are not obscured by the considerable differences of imagination and originality that exist between the individuals composing the group.

Table I demonstrates that, in one study, individual productivity varied between 5 and 94 responses. The richer records, however, proved to be multiple variations of the basic percepts. This consistency of perceptual style within a clinical group corresponds to the style of painters, which enables art experts to identify the historical period, the particular school, and the individual artist to whom an unsigned work can be attributed.

　　2. *The many possible variables of Rorschach response can be defined objectively in terms of physical determinants and of categories of contents.*

The visual percept underlying each response can be defined in terms of location, outline, kinesthesis, shading, and color that accounted for it. The meaning attributed to the percept, the "content," is significant only in respect of certain broad categories that do not involve either psychological theories or cultural value judgments. Thus, the personal preconceptions of the observer are by-passed in the description of the experimental material. This is not possible if the psychological data are obtained from interviews, biographies and primarily verbal tests, because each observer has his own focus of interest and this affects the reactions of the patient. Rorschach responses, on the other hand, are not significantly affected by the personality of the examiner (Booth, 1946a, 1946b). All this makes possible reliable control studies by other observers, who can determine objectively whether their own patients confirm previous publications or not.[4]

The psychological interpretation of the Rorschach data is indepen-dent of the fact-finding itself. Its validity can be checked against the observations of clinicians and epidemiologists.

B.   *The Difference Between the Rorschach Criteria of Somatic and
of Psychiatric Disease*

Rorschach introduced his psychodiagnostic inkblots for the specific
purpose of differentiating between neurotic, psychotic, and healthy
personalities. His tragic death in the year following the publication of
"Psychodiagnostics" prevented him from developing his method. His
numerous followers added many refinements of his basic insights but
failed to consider the possibility that subcortical systems, mediating
basic biological functions, may exercise specific influences on the
personality. Nearly all psychosomatic Rorschach research has, therefore,
endeavored to define somatic disease groups in line with Rorschach's
psychiatric criteria. Although the findings demonstrated statistical
differences, they proved to be secondary complications of the organic
diseases. They are indicative of neurotic or psychotic dynamics that are
of practical importance because they influence the prognosis. This
point has been demonstrated by excellent Rorschach studies of tuberculosis
(Lewis and Korkes, 1955) and of cancer (Shrifte, 1962). None of these
authors, however, discovered that there were *specific psychobiological
dynamics associated with the two diseases.*

The discovery of specific somatic criteria of Rorschach percepts
was the unexpected result of my early efforts (1946a) to use the
Rorschach method in the study of the personality differences between
two somatic disease groups. Clinical observation of patients suffering
from Parkinsonism, arthritis, and arterial hypertension, respectively,
had convinced me that there were significant psychological traits
associated with the predominance of tension in the locomotor system
of parkinsonian (1935) and arthritic (1937b) patients on the one hand,
and the predominance of tension in the vasomotor system on the other
hand. Since the old psychiatric scoring categories only yielded information on psychiatric superstructures, it was evident that either the Rorschach inkblots were useful only for their original purpose or else they
had to be analyzed for new criteria.

Following Freud's advice about the search for unconscious meaning
in the patient's words, I studied the Rorschach records of my patients
with "evenly poised attention," ignoring the aspects which had formerly
appeared to be the only important ones. Eventually, new dimensions in
the perception of the inkblots became obvious: the special significance
of responses co-axial with the line of symmetry, the distinction between
individualistically directed and group-directed kinesthesis, between integrating vs. disintegrating perceptual tendencies, and affinity to certain

animal perceptions (1946b).

The new perceptanalytical criteria led to the definition of two psychobiological forms of organism-environment relatednesstedness:

1. Tension in the *locomotor system* expresses the need to *control* the relationship with environmental objects;
2. Tension in the *vasomotor system* expresses the need to *adapt* itself to the given milieu.

Human beings differ genetically with respect to the relative dominance of the two needs in their behavior. On this basis one can define two types of behavior:

The *L type* is dominated by the need for action and for control of object relationships according to the personal value system which usually has been developed by identification with the dominant parent figure. Serious frustration of the need for individualistic self-assertion entails somatic disease liability in the form of reduced power of the locomotor system: arthritis and Parkinsonism.

The *V type* is dominated by the need for adaptation to the biological and social opportunities offered by the given milieu. This orientation has usually been developed by way of identification with the conforming parent figure. Friedman's (1974) type A behavior predisposing toward coronary disease exemplifies one of the disease liabilities of the V type: frustration of the need of conforming to a supporting environment entails impairment of the cardiovascular system.

The preceding results of this earlier research demonstrate that percepts of the Rorschach plates are conditioned by two levels of the personality:

1. *The level of the organism that has never been part of man's conscious experience* (Sherrington, 1941), but unconsciously influences his conscious functions. This level does not represent "common human nature," but is always individualized. Genetic factors and, to an unknown extent, intrauterine events, create different degrees of effectiveness for the many biological functions on which life depends. They are mediated through the subcortical structures of the brain and constitute the biological core of the individual. This core of the personality, particularly the dominant function, unconsciously expresses itself, on the one hand, in the form of psychobiological *behavior*, and, on the other hand, in the gestalt tendencies that the subjects manifest in their *percepts* of the ambiguously structured inkblot pictures.

2. *The level of the organism that is consciously involved in the transactions between the subject and the environment.* This level of the personality is formed by accepted and repressed postnatal experiences.

Although primarily mediated by the cortex, it also integrates the influence of the subcortical personality. The result of this process can be communicated through language.

The subject who describes his/her percepts of the 10 inkblot pictures thus provides much deeper insight into his/her psychobiological structure than has previously been realized. Originally, Rorschach percepts were analyzed only in respect of the categories of conscious psychology and of psychiatric diagnosis.

The contributions of basic biological functions to psychological processes and behavior could be objectified only by the Rorschach study of groups of individuals who, by the nature of their somatic disease, had unequivocally proved that a common biological factor had made them subject to disease of the same biological function. Clinical experience preceding the Rorschach approach (Booth, 1935, 1937b) had already indicated that organic disease occurs in the organ whose function has played a leading part in the original adjustment to life during the period of physical health. The disease manifests the fact that internal and/or external circumstances have interfered seriously with the continued healthy exercise of the preferred way of relating to the environment.

This definition of the biological foundation of the L-type and of the V-type, respectively, has made the use of Rorschach records in psychiatry considerably more precise and informative than had been the case as long as evaluations had been based on the classical method alone. In the course of the last 40 years I have administered the Rorschach to all subjects, altogether more than 1700, who consulted me with psychiatric and vocational problems. Details about the applications to psychotherapy (1960, 1963b), vocation for the ministry (1958b, 1963a), and anthropology (1963b, 1964a) have been published. Furthermore, follow-ups of many subjects confirmed the predictive value of the typology in physically healthy individuals who later in life developed somatic illness.

The above experiences led me to expect that it would be possible to investigate by means of the Rorschach method the constitutional factors involved in the epidemiology of cancer and tuberculosis.

C. *Principles of Rorschach Research in Somatic Disease*

In the course of the present investigation of cancer and tuberculosis the following principles proved to be important:

1. *The study of a genetically determined disease disposition*

requires a control group that is also characterized by a genetically determined disease.

A control group of physically healthy individuals or of accident cases would be composed of a wide variety of constitutional types, including an unknown number of candidates for the disease investigated. A control group of psychiatric cases would add the complication that psychoses and neuroses influence Rorschach perceptions in ways likely to obscure the somatic factor, and, besides, most psychiatric patients eventually develop a somatic disease.

    2. *The two clinical groups compared must have one clinical feature in common.*

This principle reduces the number of biological variables, so that the disease-related phenomena stand out most clearly; just as, in conventional psychological research projects, patients are equated for age, sex, socio-economic status, education, and intelligence. As mentioned above, in the comparison of the L-type and the V-type the factor of increased tension in the two types of motor systems was used as the equating factor. The present study of cancer and tuberculosis involved the equating principle in two different clinical dimensions:

    a) the common *disease disposition of the lungs* was used for the purpose of differentiating the dynamics of cancer and of tuberculosis;

    b) the validity of the newly found cancer criteria was tested by checking the Rorschach records of patients who suffered from *cancer in organs other than the lungs.*

    3. *Each inkblot picture must be considered separately in comparing responses of the two clinical groups.*

As explained above (p. 32), each inkblot has a specific demand character that must be taken into consideration for the proper evaluation of the percept. To give an example: the percept "fighting men" has different implications in Plate II than in Plate III, because the former is suggestive of aggressive confrontation and the latter, of conventional peaceful co-existence.

    4. *Only those types of percepts were considered significant which occurred in one group at least twice as often as in the other.*

The choice of the two-to-one ratio was made for purely practical reasons, to avoid complicated statistical calculations. The ratio establishes clearly the dynamic prevalence of the perceptual tendency in the group where it is at least twice as often expressed as in the other. Personally, I feel it is likely that the ratio reflects the effect of dominant and recessive genes, as this is the case in the Szondi Test. Some geneticists I consulted have frowned on this interpretation, but they have failed to convince me.

5. *The significance of the group-specific percepts must be confirmed by their prevalence in the individual members of the group.*

Because of the complexity of human nature and the ambiguity of the inkblot pictures, nobody produces all the percepts characteristic of his diagnostic group; but there were very few cases in which the number of specific percepts failed to exceed the number of percepts specific for the other group. The fact that most subjects responded to some of the inkblots the way members of the other group did expresses the common observation that groups representing a constitutional type are composed of individuals who respond to *most* life situations according to type but deviate in a minority of situations. The Rorschach record makes it possible to define these situations. We classify people with confidence as being conventional or unconventional characters although under certain circumstances conventional people do unconventional things, and unconventional people sometimes conform to conventions.

6. *Rorschach records obtained before the beginning of the somatic illness should conform to the pattern found in the sick and also in those recovered from the sickness.*

This last principle provides the most conclusive proof that the perceptual tendencies of a constitutional group are not due to the presence of disease. Both the disease and the response to the inkblots are manifestations of the same specific personality dynamics that in the state of health played the leading role in the subject's encounter with the environment. In view of the fact that in the last 30 years Rorschach tests have been administered to so many people for purely psychological purposes, it should not be difficult to make a follow-up study of such subjects with regard to their later organic illnesses. Even within the limitations of my private practice, so far 18 cases have come to my knowledge who developed cancer in later years.

Application of the preceding six methodological principles made it possible to establish disease-specific criteria that differentiate the perceptual tendencies of the respective predispositions for cancer and for tuberculosis in terms of numerical ratios.

The findings have two aspects:

1. The *general dynamics of the clinical group* are indicated by the total of all criteria that occur within it twice as frequently

as in the comparison group.

2. The *dynamics of the individual member of the group* are indicated by the selection of Rorschach plates in which the group-specific criteria prevail, by the individualization of the typical responses, and by other aspects of the responses that reflect complicating somatic and psychiatric factors.

Members of a clinical group vary widely in respect of the plates that elicit the disease-specific percepts. Practically all of them also perceive a minor number of plates in ways that conform with the comparison group (Tables I and II).

Since each inkblot picture symbolizes a specific life situation, the preponderance of "positive" cards expresses the fact that the individual reacts to a majority of these situations according to his disease disposition rather than according to the way of the comparison group. Disease, after all, is the response of the constitutionally dominant organ to its frustration. The somatic symptoms become the substitute for the realistic relationship between the organ and its healthy objects at the point at which either external frustration or reduced vitality has interfered beyond the level of tolerance with the individual way of life (Booth, 1946a, 1963b).

The inkblots' effectiveness in experimentally producing conditions analogous to those that cause disease is apparently due to their non-representational character. On the one hand, their dummy quality (pp. 31-33) forces the subject to perceive them as representations of realistic objects; on the other hand, *none of them makes possible a fully satisfactory identification with a realistic object.* Every Rorschach percept, considered critically, accomplishes only an incomplete and distorted approximation of the intended image, just as the sick organ exercises its psychobiological functions only in an incomplete and distorted way.

Frustrating life situations are paralleled by the frustrating perceptual demands of the inkblots. This explains the fact that the Rorschach imagery reflects in groups and in their individual members the constitutional bias in favor of specific forms of object relationships. Disease is only one of the results of the idiosyncratic interaction between subject and environment. In the state of health, the results are evident in the character of human relationships, of attitudes toward cultural values and toward nonhuman objects in work and play. In this respect, Rorschach's psychodiagnostic method validates and extends the results of L. Szondi (1948), who demonstrated that the genetic factors associated with specific psychiatric illnesses are also at the root of the choices people make in marriage, friendship, and occupation.

It is a curious fact that, in the nearly 50 years since Rorschach discovered his diagnostic instrument, so very few other psychiatrists have explored the potential of his method. It became nearly completely the domain of clinical psychologists. They, having only limited contact with medical patients, were reduced to elaborating, sometimes very ingeniously, the insights Rorschach had about the relationship between psychiatric categories and modes of visual perception. They therefore continued to report to psychiatrists on their findings within the narrow conceptual framework of psychological concepts that prevailed in the first quarter of this century, characterized by the dichotomy of psyche and soma.

Furthermore, the division of labor between psychologists and psychiatrists created among the latter the prejudice that only the psychological expert could learn something from Rorschach records. Although, unquestionably, clinical psychologists such as Zygmunt Piotrowski (1957) have made unique discoveries in the understanding of this material, the psychiatrist can learn much about his patients from studying their Rorschach imagery in light of his general knowledge of medicine and psychodynamics, and of his special knowledge of the individual patients.

Psychoanalytically trained physicians, in particular, should often find it more rewarding to interpret their patients' Rorschach records than their dreams and free associations. Technically, the administration of the test is certainly very simple and not time-consuming, and the resulting records are relatively concise and can be studied in depth by different psychiatrists more easily than tape-recordings of clinical interviews.

The direct use of the Rorschach method by psychiatrists would go far in meeting the criticism of current psychiatric practice voiced by one of our most distinguished research psychiatrists, Roy Grinker Sr. (1961), who was "shocked by the paucity of information in the hospital charts" when he was undertaking the study of phenomena of depression. He explained the lack of precise clinical descriptions as a consequence of the current psychodynamic orientation of psychiatrists. It causes the resident physician of the hospital to neglect the "graphical recording of facts"; instead, he records his inferences that "give him a feeling of closure and satisfaction."

The imagery elicited by the inkblot pictures provides a very graphic recording of the psychological situation of the patient, more graphic than mere verbal descriptions because the meaning of the visual imagery is amplified by the symbolic implications of the whole inkblot picture. The purely verbal communications between patient and physician are also more likely to be colored by situational and interpersonal factors than the imagery elicited by nonrepresentational objects, because people are generally unaware of the psychological meaning of their percepts. It is evident that much of the value of the Rorschach imagery is lost for the psychiatrist who does not look at the whole record, but reads only the inferences and selective illustrations given by the clinical psychologist. The latter's evaluation of the case may be illuminating in many respects, but he cannot convey all the potential information which may be evident to the psychiatrist who has firsthand knowledge of the patient and his Rorschach percepts.

The reluctance of psychiatrists to use the method of one of their own colleagues brings to mind the laggard acceptance of two diagnostic methods that eventually became indispensable to medical practice: Leopold Auenbrugger's work on percussion was published in 1761, but ignored until Corvisard discovered and translated it 37 years later; René T. Laënnec introduced auscultation and the stethoscope in 1818, but his innovation ran into similar resistance.

Forbes' apologetic preface to the English translation of Laënnec's work could describe equally the current attitude of psychiatrists toward the personal use of the Rorschach method. In the following quotation I have substituted only the few words [in brackets] describing inkblot pictures for those describing the stethoscope: "That [the method] will ever come into general use notwithstanding its value, I am extremely doubtful, because its beneficial application requires much time and gives a great deal of trouble to the patient and to the practitioner, because its whole hue and character are foreign, and opposed to all our habits and associations. It must be confessed that there is something even ludicrous in the picture of a grave physician proudly listening [to a patient's description of 10 inkblots] as if the disease were a living being that could communicate its condition to the sense without. Besides there is in this method a sort of bold claim and pretension to certainty and precision in diagnosis which cannot at first sight but be somewhat startling to a mind deeply versed in the knowledge and uncertainties of our art, and to the calm and cautious habits of [research] to which the English physician is accustomed." (Quotation according to René and Jean Dubos, 1952.)

The parallel between stethoscope and Rorschach test applies not only to the resistance of the profession, but also to the need for caution in drawing conclusions from these diagnostic instruments. In 1846, Thomas Addison (Harrison, 1966) warned against excessive reliance on the stethoscope, as follows: "They look upon the instrument as all sufficient;...they neglect or disdain those careful and minute inquiries which no sound and sensible physician ever fails to do, and thereby convert an invaluable auxiliary into what, in their hand at least, proves but an imperfect and treacherous substitute." The same warning, applied to the present Rorschach study of cancer, means that only careful inquiry into the epidemiological and clinical facts, as well as into the life histories of individual patients, can validate the findings resulting from use of this invaluable instrument.

On the other hand, these findings have made it possible to clarify the rationale behind the mass of seemingly unrelated and sometimes confounding facts that over the years have been accumulated by physicians, psychologists, epidemiologists, and sociologists. Once the significant dynamics had been identified in the Rorschach records, they provided the thread of Ariadne that led the way out of the Labyrinth of confusing data into the light of the unsuspected human focus of the cancer epidemic.

Later chapters (VI, VII, VIII) will trace the many ways in which Western man unconsciously created the carcinogenic milieu of the industrial age.

II

Differential Rorschach Criteria
of Cancer and Tuberculosis

A. *The Clinical Material*

The differentiating criteria of the Rorschach responses of cancer and of tuberculosis patients, respectively, were found by comparison of two clinical groups. The groups were equated for the localization of the disease process in the lungs, as well as for the usual psychological factors of age,[5] sex, literacy, socio-economic status, and severity of the illness. All the Rorschach records were obtained by the same psychologist, Dr. Lenore Korkes. They were part of her research with Dr. Nolan D.C. Lewis (1955) concerning the psychological element in the prognosis of pulmonary tuberculosis. The cancer patients were added as a control group and also in order to aid my own research project, because I had run into considerable difficulties in my attempts to obtain Rorschach records for the avowed purpose of studying the personality aspects of cancer. The irrational objections, from the side of somatically oriented physicians, to a psychodynamic study have been described previously (Booth, 1965).

The first 15 lung cancer patients (12 male, 3 female) were tested at the time of admission, before the diagnosis had been established, in order to avoid the psychological effects of the knowledge of having a very serious form of cancer. Since lung cancer is a predominantly male disease, the disproportion between the sexes was expected to reflect the underlying psychodynamic pattern of a predominantly male group.

The first 35 tuberculosis patients were all hospitalized and considered to have a poor prognosis. They were all male, in order to balance the expectedly male aspect of the lung cancer group, although tuberculosis is not a major liability of one sex.

The perceptanalytical study of the Rorschach records was undertaken *without any information on the history of the patients* beyond the fact that none in either group had undergone major surgery.

After the differential criteria of cancer and tuberculosis had been established as a result of this study, their validity was confirmed by applying them to other patients, characterized as follows:

1. *Ten unselected lung cancer cases* (9 male, 1 female) and 6 *female tuberculosis* patients (belonging to the original group of Dr. Korkes that represented poor prognosis). The records of 5 of the lung cancer patients had been obtained by E. Kuntz-Evers, M.D., in a municipal hospital in Lübeck, Germany, and those of the other 5 by myself from 4 successfully operated patients of Delafield Hospital in New York and from one patient who had consulted me in private practice on account of a depression.

2. The question had to be answered, whether the findings in the experimental groups reflected the difference between the *newly admitted* (cancer) and the *hospitalized* (tuberculosis) patients. The answer was provided by applying the Rorschach criteria to 41 tuberculosis cases (31 male, 10 female) equal to the group with unfavorable prognosis, 25 of which were fully recovered and 16 considered to have a good prognosis. Korkes and Lewis had found striking differences between the Rorschach records of these two tuberculosis groups related to good and to bad prognosis, respectively. These differences did not affect the preponderance of tuberculosis criteria over cancer criteria. As a matter of fact, because of the greater productivity of the group with good prognosis, the latter also had more tuberculosis criteria:

No.	Diagnosis	Criteria CA	TB	Proportion CA	:	TB
41	Chronic tuberculosis	196	413	1	:	2.1
41	Arrested tuberculosis	217	522	1	:	2.4

3. The findings for the lung cancer group raised the question, whether they were specific for only this clinical group or for the *disposition toward neoplastic disease in general.* This proved to be the case when the Rorschach records of patients with malignancies of other organs were examined. Fifty of the records were obtained from Dr. Miriam Shrifte, who had used them for her study of prognostic indications (1962) in 25 cases with favorable and 25 with unfavorable outcome. Again, as in the case of tuberculosis, the *Rorschach differences related to prognosis proved independent of the criteria which established the preponderance of the disease-specific criteria.* Eighteen additional cases were taken from my private practice. (The localizations of neoplasia in this group are detailed in Table I, p. 240.)

4. The scoring for cancer and tuberculosis criteria was finally applied to a group of 60 cases of *arterial hypertension* whose Rorschach records I had in my files from my earlier study of this condition (Booth, 1946b). This was done to make sure that neither the cancer proportions nor the tuberculosis proportions were characteristic of an unrelated clinical group. The results will be discussed in Section C of this chapter.

Among the cancer cases mentioned above under #1 and #3 were 12 whose records had been obtained *before there had been any evidence of neoplastic disease*, in the course of psychiatric examinations for purposes of therapy or of vocational evaluation, to two of whom the Rorschach had been administered twice. The time span between psychological testing and onset of clinical malignancy was, respectively, 25, 24, 22, 19, 17, 15, 10 (two), 9, 2, 1, and ½ years. The last-mentioned case was located in the testicle and therefore quickly discovered. The presence of the diagnostic criteria before the development of the somatic illness must be interpreted as a clear indication that they are related to *constitutional disposition and not to the disease process.*

The systematic tabulation of the results in all the categories described was concluded in 1964. Of the 93 cancer cases, only 15 had the Rorschach administered by myself—a small enough number to exclude a significant influence by the examiner. In the 10 years since then, I have seen 33 more cases in my private practice. These have confirmed the earlier findings, as have a growing number of Rorschach records shown to me by a study group of colleagues interested in my approach. Thus, there was no need to recalculate statistical frequencies for the larger number of records examined. Occasionally, in the following chapters, the larger number of records examined will be used in support of observations that occurred to me after concluding the present chapter.

B. The Perceptanalytical Criteria of Cancer and Tuberculosis

The perceptual tendencies prevailing in cancer and in tuberculosis, respectively, will be defined in the following. Some of the salient points have been illustrated with schematic sketches. It is not necessary to be trained in the psychological evaluation of Rorschach records in order to apply the present 29 pairs of cancer and tuberculosis criteria to the diagnostic scoring of Rorschach records. Psychodynamic interpretation of individual scores will be treated in the next chapter.

To obtain comparable results, these points must be observed:

1. The subject must be asked what the plate *looks* like. Some subjects try to avoid this by talking about what it makes them *think* of, particularly if they are used to "free associating."

2. It is important to remember that the present system of comparative evaluation is based on the psychological demands made by the inkblots in their *normal positions and sequence.* Patients, therefore, should be told not to rotate the cards into other positions. In case a patient disregards this instruction, his percepts should nevertheless be recorded. Although such percepts will be irrelevant for the cancer/tuberculosis score, they are apt to be psychologically revealing as attempts to escape from the type of situation symbolized by the inkblot picture in the normal position. An example for this behavior is provided most frequently by Plate VII, as described in Chapter IV.

3. For the purpose of *scoring the percepts,* it is important to *follow the given definition exactly.* This means, in particular, that percepts must be scored only if they occur in the plates for which they are described as critical. Because of the specific demand character of each Rorschach plate, the same type of percept will have a different diagnostic meaning if it occurs on different plates; for example, the same type of kinesthesis is typical for tuberculosis in Plate I and for cancer in Plate VIII. To give another instance: it is typical for cancer to interpret Plate X as one whole scene or object, but in Plates I, V, and VII the diagnostic significance of the same percept

does not change, whether the percept applies to the whole inkblot or only to the axial area as far as cancer criteria are concerned.

4. With respect to the scoring of the records, it is important to remember that the only basis is the *occurrence of a certain criterion, not the number* of percepts satisfying the same criterion. Repetitive expressions of the same basic percept belong in the category of the conscious and subconscious psychological reactions that are mainly transacted on the cortical level of the nervous system. On the level of the subcortical functions involved in somatic diseases, the only important point is whether a certain *quality* of perception occurs.

5. For the evaluation of the whole record, not only the total number of critical percepts is important, but also *the number of Rorschach plates in which either* cancer or tuberculosis criteria prevail. Since each plate represents a specific existential situation, it is important to determine how many the subject reacts to in accordance with one or the other disease tendency. This will eliminate from the final clinical score those plates that elicited *no critical percepts and also those in which the contrasting criteria were equally* represented.

For the purpose of differentiating the basic dynamics of cancer and of tuberculosis, it is irrelevant which Rorschach plates the final scores were derived from. For understanding the *individual patient*, however, it is important to consider the specific plates to which he or she reacts, according to the clinical diagnosis. Some of the following descriptions of criteria may appear excessively detailed, particularly to persons used to the current scoring methods of clinical psychologists. There are, however, quite specific meanings that will become clear in the next chapter, which will go into the psychological interpretation of the 29 contrasting pairs of criteria.

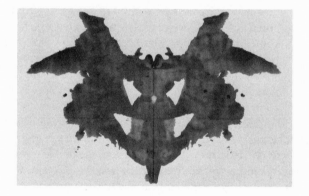

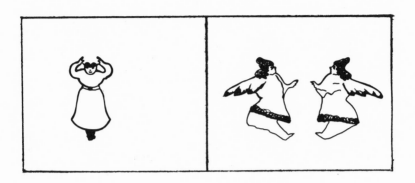

PLATE I

CANCER	TUBERCULOSIS

1.

The *axial* area is emphasized as the dynamic center of a warm-blooded organism other than a bat, as two people in close contact, or as center of inanimate forces; e.g., "exploding tank," "iron pieces in magnetic field."

The *lateral* areas are interpreted as two organisms *seen as a pair*; e.g., angels, birds, dogs.

2.

Kinesthesis indicates *intention*; e.g., claws ready to grasp, birds about to take off.

Kinesthesis indicates *action*; e.g., flying, dancing. (Flying bats and butterflies were not included in the score because it seems an easily suggested response. Actually, it occurs only in the TB group.)

3.

The content implies *hiding*; e.g., "a mask" or "a person masquerading as a bat."

The content has *exhibitionistic* character; e.g., "exotic headgear," "butterfly in a display case," "a bat larger than a normal bat."

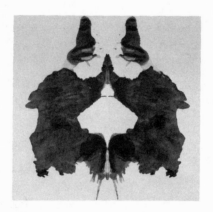

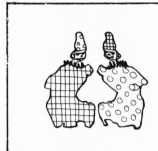 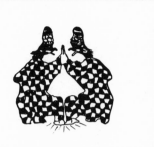

PLATE II

CANCER	TUBERCULOSIS

1.

The vertical axis (whole or in part) is co-axial with a *natural object,* e.g., butterfly, goat head, volcano, sun. (Isolated sex organs are not scored.)

The vertical axis (whole or in part) is co-axial with an *artifact* ("monument," "spinning top") or an anatomical object, e.g., pelvic bone or isolated sex organ.

2.

The two large lateral areas are described as human beings or animals, either *unrelated* to each other ("two witches doing nothing") *or pursuing self-assertive purposes* ("two bears fighting" or "eating").

The two large lateral areas are described as human beings or animals engaged in a *positive social relationship*, e.g., dancing, toasting, playing together.

3.

The content of the *kinesthesis is seen as unequivocal.*

The content of any *kinesthesis is equivocal*, e.g., the bears are either dancing or fighting.

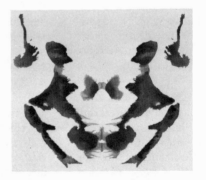

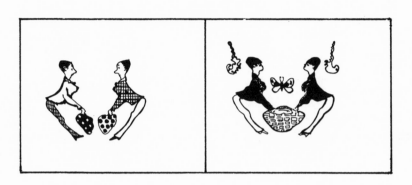

PLATE III

CANCER

1.

The popular human figures are described as either *unrelated or as pursuing self-assertive purposes* (cf. Plate II, 2) e.g., each carrying his own bundle, or fighting for the object between them.

2.

Contentincludes*non-domesticated warm-blooded* animals, very often birds.

3.

The colored areas are *not interpreted.*

4.

Kinesthesis of the popular human figures is *unequivocal* (cf. Plate II, 3).

TUBERCULOSIS

The popular human beings are seen as *socially interacting* (cf. Plate II, 2) e.g., lifting an object together, or dancing together.

Content includes *domesticated,* warm-blooded animals, e.g., dogs, chickens, ducks.

The colored details are *interpreted.*

Kinesthesis of the popular human figures is *equivocal* (cf. Plate II, 3).

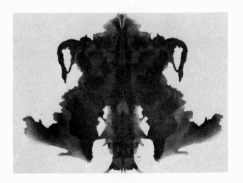

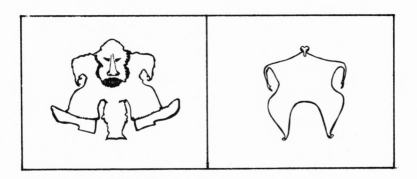

PLATE IV

CANCER	TUBERCULOSIS

1.

The whole inkblot suggests the image of an *intact, warm-blooded organism,* a *tree* or a *flower.* (*Bat* is not included because not discriminating).

The whole or the major part (see illustration) of the inkblot suggests either an organism which is *crippled or decayed,* or parts of an organism in this state, e.g., animal skin. (The *unqualified* latter response is not scored under this heading because it is not discriminating.)

2.

Content of responses to any area refers to *undomesticated warm-blooded* animals other than "bat" or "bear."

Content of responses to any area refers to a *domesticated* animal, e.g., cowhide.

3.

Content refers to *large size* or to *aggression,* e.g., "picture of a monster to scare people," "hunter shooting a bear" (edge detail).

Content refers to small size, weakness or looking down, e.g., "looking down on the smashed head of a bull."

4.

Content does *not* refer to hiding, clothing, or some supporting background.

Content refers to *hiding, clothing or a support* not represented by inkblot, e.g., "bat nailed to barn door."

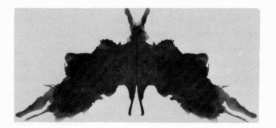

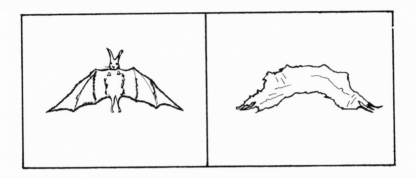

PLATE V

CANCER

The whole or the *axial area* is seen as a *whole warm-blooded organism* other than a bat, e.g., eagle, winged rabbit, two people embracing, a person masquerading as a bat. As in Plate IV the content of the responses tends to refer to a more powerful organism than the popular bat or butterfly.

TUBERCULOSIS

The whole or the *axial area* is seen either as an artifact (airplane, bridge), as life ended (split carcass, decaying tree trunk) or threatened (bird caught between rocks, deer going off between bushes, Madame Butterfly).

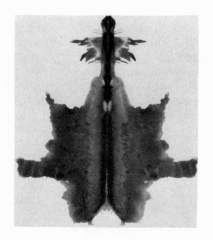

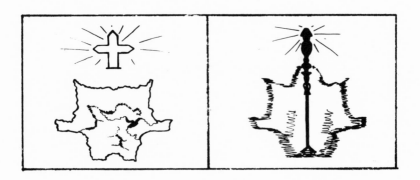

PLATE VI

CANCER	TUBERCULOSIS
1.	
The whole inkblot or the larger bottom areas are given some interpretation, but the "animal skin" either is missed totally or is qualified; e.g., "two halves of skins lying together," "forepart has been cut off."	The popular "animal skin" is seen without the qualifications described for the cancer group.
2.	
Both top and bottom areas are interpreted, but as *unrelated* objects; e.g., "totem post" *and* "Janus head"; "cross" *and* "relief map" (illustrated).	Both top and bottom areas are interpreted as individual, but *interrelated*, objects; e.g., "cross overlooking a piece of ground," "floor lamp on a rug" (illustrated).
3.	
The animal skin is seen as *not related* to an imagined background (cf. Plate IV, 4).	The animal skin is seen as *related* to a background that is not suggested by a part of the inkblot; e.g., "spread over stones to dry," or "in front of a fireplace."

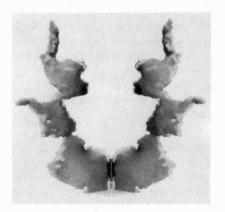

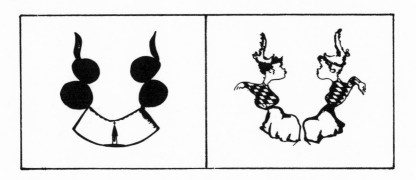

PLATE VII

CANCER	TUBERCULOSIS

1.

The *whole inkblot*, the *axial area,* or the *axial white space* is seen as a solid object; e.g., an atoll, a necklace (illustrated), a steeple illustrated), or a bust of George Washington (upside down in white space). All these responses *ignore the suggestion of two autonomous but interrelated organisms.*

The *lateral areas* are interpreted, either as paired or as independent figures. If the bottom detail is mentioned only as an adjunct to the lateral details (e.g., as "busts standing on *some sort* of a base"), this is not scored as "cancer type" response. The latter score would be added if the bottom detail were more differentiated; e.g., "seesaw on which two children are sitting."

2.

The whole inkblot is seen as a group of *six objects of the same kind*; e.g., heads of people, kernels of nuts, shells on the beach, fried shrimp, cookies.

The response implies incompleteness, *disintegration*, or instability; e.g., a one-legged dancer (upside down), melting snow, precariously balanced acrobats or stones.

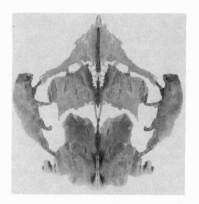

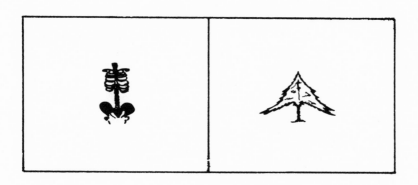

PLATE VIII

CANCER	TUBERCULOSIS
1.	
Axial areas are seen as anatomical or pathological structures.	Axial areas are seen as natural objects; e.g., rock, mountain, live tree, or animal of any kind.
2.	
The popular "animals" in the latteral details are seen in *free action*; e.g., climbing, prowling, walking.	The lateral "animals" are either *not seen in any action* or the action has a *strained* character; e.g., "hanging on," "trying to escape from the fire below," "as if going to leap."
3.	
The responses are *unqualified*.	The responses are *tentative*; e.g., "I guess it must be a tree," "a lamb *or* a buffalo *or* a bear."

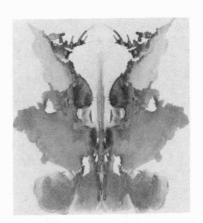

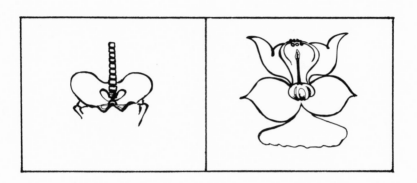

PLATE IX

CANCER	TUBERCULOSIS

1.

Responses to the whole or to the axial part of the inkblots connote *disintegration of organic forms:* anatomy, isolated sex organs, buttocks, disease, dying flower, uprooted plant, non-objective art, A-bomb.

Responses to the whole or to the axial parts of the inkblot involve *life:* plants, animals, *flowing* water, sky, sun.

2.

The spiky orange details on top are either not interpreted at all, or are given non-aggressive meaning, e.g., carrot.

The spiky orange details on top are given aggressive meaning, e.g., closing mechanism of carnivorous plant, claws, spitting dragons.

3.

Human and animal forms are seen without kinesthetic interpretations.

Human and animal forms are seen kinesthetically, e.g., Icarus, children moving balloons up and down, mountain climbers.

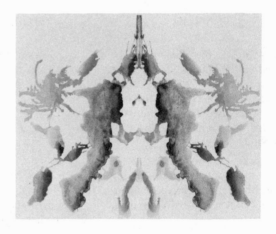

Reproduced by permission of Verlag Hans Huber, Bern, Switzerland
The original was produced with color

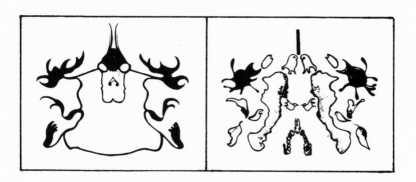

PLATE X

CANCER	TUBERCULOSIS

1.

At least one response intends to cover the *whole inkblot*; e.g., a garden scene, a showcase of insects.

Only details are interpreted, without reference to the whole.

2.

Details usually seen as separate objects *are fused into larger units*; e.g., "a fantastic beetle" (illustrated), "an orchid," "an ornate brooch," "iridescent oil film on a puddle," are whole responses. Partial fusions are exemplified by the combination of the "rabbit head" and "two green worms" a "horseshoe," "tongs," or a "mandible," or adding to the popular "blue crab" the adjacent green as its "big claw."

The responses involve *disintegration*; e.g., "a body riddled with disease," "the blue spots in the middle show where the testicles were," the popular "yellow dogs" have no hind legs. In defense against this dismaying percept, the areas of the same color frequently are divided into smaller units; e.g., the usual "blue crab" into "two bugs fighting," or "a nest in a tree."

3.

The axial top gray spot is either *not interpreted at all*, or interpreted only in reduced form; e.g., "feelers of bug" (illustrated).

The axial part of the top is interpreted as a *solid object*; e.g., "Eiffel Tower," "pole," "Spinal column."

C.   The Quantitative Findings

The *relative* frequencies of the criteria for cancer and for tuberculosis, respectively, were found to differ in the four clinical groups, as follows:

Lung cancer	1 : 0.37
Other Cancers	1 : 0.47
Arterial Hypertension	1 : 0.81
Pulmonary tuberculosis	1 : 2.28

The results prove that the most impressive differences were found between the two original experimental groups. They confirm the importance of limiting the somatic variables in psychosomatic research (cf. Chapter I, C). A detailed background for the above figures is found in Tables I—III and Fig. I (p. 240ff).

The findings in the cases of arterial hypertension indirectly validate the concept of pathogenesis that has provided the theoretical basis for the present research: that in case of marked preponderance of one specific functional system over a counterbalancing functional system, the reality adjustment of the organism is apt to break down in the area of the dominant function. This principle was first discovered by Jung (1923) in his study of psychological types and confirmed for somatic diseases in my study of arthritis, Parkinsonism, and arterial hypertension (Booth, 1946b). It is evident that the arterial hypertension group is characterized by a fair balance of cancer and tuberculosis tendencies, making the likelihood of either disease remote in this group.

Closer examination of the individual cases in this group, furthermore, confirmed that the proportion of cancer—tuberculosis criteria has clinical significance:

1. The slight predominance of cancer criteria is due to the fact that 11 patients had the critical cancer ratio of 1 : 0.5 but only two had the tuberculosis ratio of 1 : 2. The incidence of 18 percent cancer-prone and 3 percent tuberculosis-prone individuals corresponds approximately to the epidemiological data of the population in the 1930's, when the data were collected.

2. Examination of the case histories at the Rockefeller Institute which had provided the material for the Rorschach study of arterial hypertension (Booth, 1946a) revealed that, of the patients with *"cancer scores,"* one had been successfully

operated for a leiomyosarcoma of the stomach three years before the testing, another had been found to have a shadow in his chest x-ray suggesting lymphosarcoma or Hodgkins disease. When he was re-examined after a few weeks, the shadow had disappeared, leading to the interpretation that it had been caused by an abnormally radiation-sensitive tumor of the type described by Tilden C. Everson and Warren H. Cole in their study of spontaneous regression in cancer (1966). One of the patients with a *"tuberculosis score,"* incidentally, was at that time suspected of having tuberculosis of one kidney, but during the period of follow-up the diagnosis was not clarified.

Some of the implications of the tabulations of the *frequency range of cancer and tuberculosis criteria* (Table I) may be pointed out specifically:

1. Disease is correlated, not with a high number of criteria specific for the group, but *only with their relative preponderance* over the criteria of the contrasting group.
2. Not one of the records in any of the four clinical groups included all of the 29 criteria for either cancer or tuberculosis.

Comparison between clinical and Rorschach diagnosis (Tables II and III) calls for the following observations:

1. *Lung cancer:* the complete agreement of clinical and Rorschach diagnosis is the result of the experimental design. Only those criteria were used which provided unequivocal results for all 25 cases. (The 26th additional case came in later as one of the 50 cases of Dr. Shrifte.)
2. *Other cancers:* clinical and Rorschach diagnosis agreed in 95.5 percent of the cases, on the basis of a count of all individual criteria, and in 97 percent of all cases, comparing the number of plates in which cancer criteria prevailed over tuberculosis criteria. The fact that in this group the margin of cancer over tuberculosis criteria was smaller than in the lung cancer group proves that in those other localizations additional perceptual tendencies are expressed, which are related to the dynamics of the diseased organ system. This is apparent from the higher percentage of percepts unrelated to either neoplastic or tuberculous conditions of the lungs (see Table IV, p. 240).
3. *Tuberculosis:* clinical and Rorschach diagnosis agreed in 87 percent of the cases, on the basis of a count of all individual

criteria, and in 92.7 percent of all cases, comparing the number of plates in which tuberculosis criteria prevailed over cancer criteria. The fact that a small percentage of tuberculosis cases showed a tendency toward neoplasia bears out the many clinical observations on record that former tuberculosis patients sometimes develop lung cancer late in life (Barnes, 1960; Collas, 1964; Schwartz, 1960; Westergren, 1959).

The tabulations of the *diagnostic scores for each individual Rorschach plate* make clear that within the clinical groups considerable *individual variety* is found in respect of the conditions under which the pathogenic responses are produced. This variability, illustrated by Figure 1 and Table I, expresses itself in the following forms:

1. The number of plates to which the patient responds *in conformity with his clinical condition* ranges between 2 and 8. The average of "positive" responses in cancer was 6; in tuberculosis, 5.

2. Most patients respond to *some* plates with percepts *characteristic of the other clinical group.* In cancer, the number of plates eliciting TB-type criteria ranges between 0 and 5, and the same range was found in tuberculosis. The average of plates eliciting deviant scores was 1.1 in cancer and 1.7 in tuberculosis.

3. Patients respond to one or more Rorschach plates in a manner that is *not characteristic for either* cancer or tuberculosis. This results from one of the following circumstances:

    b) none of the responses falls under any of the definitions given for the tuberculosis criteria; e.g., "bat" in Plates I and V, "bear skin" in Plate IV, "clouds" in Plate VII.

The occurrence of variants within the range of the diagnostic score, as cited above, is consistent with the clinical experience that in many respects patients suffering from the same disease are very unlike each other. Some of the differences are due to the fact that different life situations are pathogenic for them; other differences are rooted in dimensions of the personality that have nothing to do with the dynamics of cancer and tuberculosis. For instance, cancer criterion #1 of Plate III is met by each of the percepts, "two people carrying their bundles" and "two people fighting for the object between them," but the social attitudes expressed are very different.

Since the present monograph is confined to the dynamics all cancer patients have in common, Rorschach percepts are discussed here only insofar as they are pertinent to this theme. A full Rorschach evaluation of individual patients involves many other perceptanalytical categories, which have been established by Rorschach and his followers and which are presented very clearly in Piotrowski's "Perceptanalysis" (1957).

III

The Psychological Interpretation
of the Findings

As briefly mentioned in Chapter I, Rorschach designed the series of inkblot pictures with the intention of varying their abstract aesthetic qualities. While doing this, he created 10 representational works of art that symbolize specific existential situations. In what follows, the meanings of these situations will be described for each plate separately as background for the discussion of the specific significance of the criteria predominating in each of the two disease types.

A. The Objective Gestalt of the Ten Inkblots and the Percepts of Cancer and Tuberculosis Patients

PLATE I

Rorschach (1921) planned that this inkblot should make different kinds of percepts equally easy: static form, kinesthesis, responses to the whole and to larger or smaller details. Georg A. Roemer later pointed out (1937) that the inkblot also provides equal opportunities for perceiving it as a "primitive whole" (e.g., "bat"), as two halves (e.g., "two angels"), or as a "combination whole" (e.g., "two angels carrying the person in the middle to heaven"). Furthermore, the central figure can be seen as either one or two persons, as an animal, or as an object.

This first inkblot of the series faces the subject with an experience analogous to the experience of *being born* into a situation radically different from anything previously experienced. The basic gestalt is that of a lower humanlike figure overtopped by larger lateral areas, a configuration suggestive of the infant emerging from the body of the mother. Since the lateral areas also easily suggest human figures, the resulting picture is suggestive of the famous antique relief usually captioned "The Birth of Venus," which shows two female figures aiding a central female figure. The movement of the latter is ambiguous and fits the interpretation of this work, instead, as a scene from the myth of Persephone, the daughter of the grain goddess Demeter, who spends the warm season with her mother on earth and the cold season in the underworld.[6] This antique symbolization of birth, death and resurrection was certainly known to Rorschach, the son of an art teacher, who had seriously considered art as his vocation before he decided to become a physician (Ellenberger, 1954). The great originality of his inkblot pictures and his perceptive interpretations of forms and colors warrant the assumption that he was not misled by the popular misnomer of the relief, which reflects the fact that people would rather think of love than of the basic polarity of life and death. The conclusion that the relief inspired the beginning of the series is supported by the fact that the concluding plate of the series is very clearly inspired by the Greek mythological image of death (p. 109 & ff.).

The balanced, manifold possibilities inherent in the first inkblot are analogous to the situation into which the subject was born. In the first months of life the innate vitality and the genetic endowment determine the effect of the first environmental constellation on the psychological development of the infant and leave their imprint on the adult personality. This explains the fact that individual percepts of Plate I are often directly or indirectly associated with childhood experiences (Booth, 1958b). Ferencz Merei describes (1953) the demand character of the first inkblot as: "The presenting of one's own self. The inner situation." Certainly, as far as the external situation is concerned the sight of the first inkblot creates the experience of a momentary loss of the familiar object world. The resulting anxiety forces the subject to fall back on his inner world and to create from the nonrepresentational inkblot those images that have personal meaning.

THE CANCER CRITERIA

1. The *emphasis on the axial area* can be interpreted on the basis of similar findings in my previous (1946b) study of

arthritis and Parkinson patients, the locomotor personality type, to be referred to in future as the *L type* (see Chapter I, B, p. 36). The axial emphasis expresses an individualistic attitude in facing the world. The values of the subject are his primary concern; the values of the environment are of secondary importance.

In 1956, Lawrence LeShan and R.E. Worthington demonstrated that cancer patients were characterized by desperate clinging to a circumscribed form of object relationships. When they felt they had lost their object without hope of retrieving it, they developed cancer. My own observations (1965, 1969b) led to a more precise definition of the psychodynamics involved. The desperate attitude proved to be the result of inadequate mothering in the first year of life, which caused strong fixations on pregenital, possessive object-relationships and prevented the development of psychosexual maturity. Furthermore, it became apparent that cancer-prone individuals sought self-fulfillment in the sphere of the psychobiological function—whether it was sex, breathing, eating, or whatever—that was dominant in their genetic endowment. Neoplasia developed in the organ that mediated the dominant function, and thus represented the regressive expression of the original striving for self-fulfillment.

This pathological process is a manifestation of a much-neglected aspect of the evolution of life. As the zoologist Adolf Portmann demonstrated (1956), the enormous profusion of differentiated forms and color patterns throughout the animal kingdom, from protozoa to man, can be explained only partly as the result of survival needs. There is also an autonomous striving for differentiation of *self-representation* that at times conflicts with survival needs; e.g., the antlers of the Irish elk and the descent of the testicles in land-living mammals. Disease does not put an end to the striving for self-representation, it merely means regression to a lesser degree of biological differentiation. Cancer cells retain some of the qualities of the organ of origin, just as the structural changes of other diseases are regressive self-representations, as I have pointed out for vascular disease, arthritis, and Parkinsonism (1946a, 1946b, 1948, 1975).

Having described cancer patients as individualistic, like the L type of personality, and disease as regressive manifestation of frustrated object-control, an explanation may be called for of why the L type does not develop malignancy in response to frustration. The difference is due to the fact that the cancer disposition is created at the very beginning of extrauterine life when the infant struggles for survival, prior to the development of object relationships; specifically, prior to the development of the locomotor system. Practically all malignancies originate in organs that already function at birth. The locomotor system becomes effective very slowly in the course of the first two years. This ontogenetic difference is consistent with the fact that cancer constitutes a threat to life, whereas arthritis and Parkinsonism, the two main diseases of the locomotor system, are generally compatible with a normal life span.

2. The predominance of percepts implying locomotor *intentions* differentiates cancer patients from those belonging to the tuberculosis type and the L types. This finding is in keeping with the role of self-representation in cancer. Intention movements, as we know from ethology (Tinbergen, 1955; Lorenz, 1966), are forms of self-representation. Their effectiveness depends on the display of the inner disposition of the organism and not on physical power (Masserman and Sievers, 1944). Infants certainly communicate their moods through their locomotor system long before they are capable of purposeful action.

3. The frequency of percepts implying *hiding* (50 percent of all lung cancer and 33 percent of all cervix cancer cases) seems to contradict the preceding manifestations of the primary need for self-representation in this group. Actually, self-representation serves the *inner* needs of the organism, and secrecy, therefore, protects self-fulfillment against outside interference. The phenomenon has been clinically confirmed by many observers (e.g., Abrams and Finesinger, 1953; Kissen, 1963) and is natural enough, considering the background of mutilated self-development in the very beginning of the lives of these subjects (LeShan and Worthington, 1956; Booth, 1969b). More will be said about this in Chapter VII, B.

The defensive self-concealment of cancer patients sets them apart, not only from the tuberculosis group, but also from the 120 patients on whom my differentiation of the L type and the V (for Vasomotor) type is based (Booth, 1946b). Only one of those 120 produced a "hiding" percept: a hypertensive man who was concealing a huge gambling debt from his wife. Most L and V patients are conditioned to living without need for concealment: L patients, because they identify with the dominant parent and feel righteous; and V patients, because they identify with the conforming parent and endeavor to meet the expectations of their social environment (Booth, 1946b).

As mentioned in the Introduction, cancer patients share their genetic predisposition with tuberculosis patients but have developed a different disease liability because of early infantile conditioning. This is evident from the different psychological dynamics found to prevail in tuberculosis patients.

THE TUBERCULOSIS CRITERIA

1. The prevailing percept of the lateral details as paired implies that, in this group, interpersonal relationships are experienced as existentially more important than individualistic self-expression. Apparently, life began with an adequate dyadic experience of the mother relationship (Spitz, 1965; Balint, 1968). As pointed out above, the individualistic percept of cancer patients suggests primacy of the survival instinct.
2. The "basic trust" (Erikson, 1963) engendered by the dyadic infantile experience favored spontaneity of behavior, whereas their infantile insecurity made cancer patients wary of acting according to their impulses.
3. Self-display is a normal part of infantile communication, but cancer patients learned as infants that communication is risky.

The percepts of Plate I illustrate the infantile background of the epidemiological fact that since 1850 a steadily increasing proportion of the genetically tuberculosis-prone fifth of the population has become cancer prone. Tuberculosis-prone individuals need an abnormal amount of affection and have been increasingly traumatized by the depersonalization of infant care which made breast feeding obsolete (Booth, 1969b). This genetic factor is emphasized in order to obviate the possible misunderstanding that depersonalized nursing, as such, should be considered a cancerogenic factor. Eighty percent of the population has proven immune to the host of cancerogenic agents that are currently blamed, and others that animal research is likely to add to the list. The liability of 20 percent is bad enough and the practical aspects of the problem will be discussed in Chapters VIII, B, and IX.

PLATE II

Rorschach planned to introduce the emotional shock effect of the color red. Furthermore, he made it difficult to separate the red from the black, by partial blending of the two areas. The configuration induces kinesthesis more easily than the preceding plate does. In addition, a conspicuous white space occupies the center of the inkblot picture.

This plate is most effective as a test of the reaction to direct interpersonal confrontation. It achieves this function by the following features:

1. The projection of one integral organism is practically impossible. For the person anxious to deal individualistically with situations, there are inescapably *two sides* confronting each other, unless major parts of the configuration are disregarded.
2. In the context of two human or animal figures facing each other at close range, the striking red color easily suggests blood and, by implication, an aggressive encounter.
3. The merging of red and black makes it difficult to avoid the emotional stimulation of the red by concentrating on the "rational" black alone.
4. The white space offers opportunities for fantasy escape from the challenge of close interpersonal confrontation.

Merei (1953) felt that this card brings out the relationship between sexuality and affectivity. This formulation applies in some cases, but it does not distinguish clearly between the primary and the secondary aspects of the situation symbolized. Primary is the *threat of disintegration as the consequence of conflict:* disintegration of a social relationship, disintegration of the body itself. Coping with this threat may take very different forms; e.g., overt or latent sexual excitement, rage or humor, sociability or withdrawal.

THE CANCER CRITERIA

1. The need for individual self-expression leads to the tendency to endow axial areas of the inkblot and/or the white space with the quality of life. These "monolithic" solutions suggest that the subject prefers limited self-expression to involvement in a close interpersonal relationship.
2. If two human or animal figures are recognized, they tend to be perceived either as self-contained or as fighting each other.
3. The tendency to perceive only one kinesthetic possibility indicates that great anxiety for individualistic self-expression makes the subject unaware of all other possibilities. This

inflexibility accounts for the "brittle object relationships" of cancer patients that was first observed by Evans (1926), explained by LeShan and Worthington (1956), and traced to its infantile origin in 1969 (Booth, 1969b) (see Chapters V-VII).

THE TUBERCULOSIS CRITERIA

1. The singular axial areas are experienced as dead objects, in keeping with the "consumptive" reaction to an existence without close interpersonal relationship.
2. Positive social relationships of the two human or animal figures are perceived, in keeping with the symbiotic needs of tuberculosis patients.
3. The patients do not attach themselves to one particular form of relatedness, but feel free to reach out for new opportunities. This flexibility is their defense against the threat of destruction by loss of a love object. Defense in the form of aggression is very rare.

This last point may be illustrated by Ebstein's list (1932) of 115 famous tuberculosis victims. Although it was the author's intention to demonstrate the great variety of personalities, and although tuberculosis has been one of the most frequently occurring diseases in European history, the only name associated with military achievement was that of Attila, king of the Huns. Even if the medical diagnosis made in 453 A.D. should be accepted as correct, the case would not change the conclusion that aggressiveness is rarely associated with consumption.

From the preceding observations, the conclusion can be drawn that tuberculosis patients have personalities that favor recovery. Even when seriously ill, they continue to seek affectionate relationships that might compensate for their pathogenic loss. Cancer patients experience the disease as confirmation of their lifelong conviction that they cannot expect affectionate support from others. This makes them liable to miss opportunities for finding new, healing relationships. This problem will be discussed in the chapter on therapy (see Chapter IX).

PLATE III

To Rorschach, the most important features of this inkblot were that the red areas are clearly separated from the black areas and that the black areas elicit, more easily than any of the other plates, kinesthetic percepts of human figures.

Plate III specifically tests the reaction of the subject to a *conventional social situation.* This function is achieved by the following:

1. The black areas are easily perceived as two human beings facing each other. They are not in direct physical contact, as was the case in Plate II, but are nevertheless close enough to each other to allow for percepts of any number of different forms of relationship. The obviousness of the human figures and their distance serve the same purpose as social conventions: the facilitation of interpersonal relationships that do not demand deeper personal involvement.

2. The "human figures" have a sexually ambiguous character. Either sex can identify with them. The secondary role of gender clues is in keeping with the suggestion of a conventional social situation in which the sex of the individuals is evident but is not given overt sexual expression.

3. The black area in the center lends itself to a great variety of interpretations. It can be perceived as an implement of cooperative activity, or as an object for which two rivals contend, or as two objects handled by two individuals independently, etc. Furthermore, the central area may be either completely ignored or perceived as one or more objects functionally unrelated to the "human figures."

4. The red color, with its implication of aggression and strong emotion, is clearly separated from the "human figures." This makes it easy to keep aggression "in the back of one's head" and to avoid "seeing red." Social conventions serve the same purpose.

5. The red color areas are given outlines, which makes it easy to interpret only their forms and to ignore the emotional implications of red; e.g., the details in the back of the "heads" seen as "monkeys," the center detail as a "butterfly" or a "bow tie." On the other hand, the color may predominate in percepts such as "blood" or "gay decorations." Obviously, the red may also be ignored as "meaningless blotches" or as "meant to confuse the patient."

Merei (1953) found the achievement of the popular solution (#1) to be critical for schizoid personalities. Thus, he singled out the group that was most limited in capacity to function on the strength of social conventions, in contrast to cancer patients, who very rarely are schizophrenic (Lewis, 1924; Rassidakis, 1974).

THE CANCER CRITERIA

1. The kinesthetic percept of the human figures indicates that cancer patients pursue individualistic purposes within the conventional structure of society.
2. The predominance of percepts of *undomesticated animals* over those of domesticated ones suggests that these patients rely on their individual survival instincts rather than on conventional "social adjustment." This is most obvious in those cases in which the popular human figures are perceived as animals, each time undomesticated ones; e.g., ostriches.
3. The tendency to ignore the colored areas suggests a strong inclination to avoid emotional situations.
4. As in Plate II, limitation to one kinesthetic percept of the human figure indicates that even in a conventional social situation cancer patients act as individuals who feel that their opportunities for object relationships are limited.

It may be concluded that cancer patients tend to display in their interpersonal relationships a rigid, individualized attitude even when the situation is conventional, not only when it is threatening (cf. Plate II). There are two important consequences of this commitment to a rigid self-image maintained against all environmental demands and opportunities for adjustments and inner changes:

The *favorable* consequence of their intense involvement in limited object-relationships makes them generally realistic and successful in their pursuits until either the devitalizing effect of age or external events deprive them of continued enjoyment of their individualistic life styles.

The *dangerous* consequence of the brittle rigidity of their object-relationships is that they experience even normal changes as irretrievable losses; e.g., that children become independent, that marriage partners mature, that they reach the limit of success in their field of endeavor.

Two historical personalities may illustrate the object-relationships of cancer personalities:

1. The late Senator Robert A. Taft Sr. was characterized (Robbins, 1954) as one whom neither "public abuse [nor] private pressure could pry loose from an opinion. Quite literally he was a man who would rather be right than President." This point was substantiated in 1952 when the Republican Party, shy of Taft's uncompromising personal integrity, nominated the conformist Dwight D. Eisenhower as its presidential candidate. Four and a half months after Eisenhower's inauguration, Taft developed the first symptoms of a cancer which had

metastasized rapidly from a minute primary lung cancer and which killed him eight weeks later. President Eisenhower's subsequent medical history demonstrated that he was a cardiovascular type. (Cf. Chapter VII, B, and the discussion of Plate VIII in this chapter.)

2. Wilhelm C. Roentgen, whom I knew well, particularly during the last years of his life, had lived nearly exclusively as a dedicated physicist. In his last years he had been depressed because he had failed to make any major contributions to experimental physics since he discovered the x-rays in 1895. Furthermore, his field had become dominated by the spectacular advances of theoretical physics which he found increasingly difficult to follow. By 1923, he also found himself socially isolated and morally offended by the beginning political corruption of German academic life evident in an attempt of colleagues to draw him into their campaign against "the Jewish theory of relativity." He died that year of cancer of the rectum.

THE TUBERCULOSIS CRITERIA

1. The contents of the kinesthetic percepts indicate that tuberculosis patients experience *participation in social situations* as the basis for self-fulfillment, making the pursuit of individual purpose a subordinate concern.
2. The predominance of percepts of *domesticated animals* is consistent with the fact that tuberculosis-prone subjects, like domesticated animals, depend for survival on their human environment rather than on their powers of individual self-assertion. Tuberculosis is most deadly among the socio-economically disadvantaged members of the population.
3. The spontaneous responsiveness to the red areas of the inkblot is evidence that tuberculosis patients readily involve themselves in the emotional aspects of a social situation, even when it is made easy to ignore them.
4. As with Plate II, the perception of multiple potential meanings of the same area of the inkblot indicates that tuberculosis patients enjoy a feeling of freedom in relating to their environment.

All these criteria suggest a common denominator of the tuberculosis-prone group: the need for interpersonal involvement, which predominates over the need for individualistic, idiosyncratic object-relationships.

On the biological level, the group is dominated by *symbiotic* needs. In recent decades, under the influence of Erich Fromm (1947), "symbiotic" has acquired among psychologists the pejorative meaning of "parasitical." Actually, symbiosis designates the *mutually beneficial* interdependence of different species of plants and animals, as exemplified by the relationship between man and the bacterial population of his bowels (Dubos, 1965; Thomas, 1974). Only if the living conditions become unfavorable for one or the other symbiotic partner will disease develop.

In the case of the relationship between man and the mycobacterium tuberculosis, until the beginning of the present century populations were regularly exposed to the infection, but the vast majority developed adequate defenses. Only in the tuberculosis-prone fifth of the population (Cherry, 1924, 1925) would immunity break down when these persons' dominant needs for affectionate relationships became frustrated (Wittkower, 1949; Kissen, 1958).

The psychosexual significance of infectious disease was originally observed by Viktor von Weizsaecker (1934) and Rudolf Bilz (1936) in a series of cases of acute tonsillitis. The illness developed at the point at which intense sexual desire was frustrated. Bacteria took the place of the human partner, symbiotic interaction was displaced from the genital to the oral organ, and the interpersonal crisis weakened the immune defenses.

This regression from the conscious interpersonal to the unconscious intercellular level adumbrates the earliest stage of the evolution of sexuality, where two amoebae could revive themselves by close contact without fusion, millions of years before the continuity of life was to be secured uniquely by the encounter of a male with a female cell. The dramatic happenings in the case of acute infection are mentioned in this discussion of tuberculosis because the chronic course of the disease makes the connection between psychosexual frustration and the cellular process less evident. Nevertheless, until Robert Koch irrefutably demonstrated the bacterium in 1882, the emotional factor in tuberculosis had been considered so evident that all earlier discoverers of the infectious factor (Dubos and Dubos, 1952) were ignored.

The strong symbiotic motivation of the tuberculosis-prone personality type explains not only why frustration causes such persons to regress to the level of the infectious process, but also why, before the discovery of drug therapy, they so often recovered when they found a new opportunity for returning to an emotionally satisfactory interpersonal relationship.

The greater facility of tuberculosis patients for establishing new object relationships has, however, also a *negative aspect* which has been noted by many observers: Because symbiotic relatedness, as such, is more important for this group than the preservation of the rigid life style typical of cancer patients, tuberculosis patients are likely to form affectionate relationships of an inferior and eventually destructive nature. This has led to moralizing evaluations of their characters as unstable and irresponsible. *Institutional treatment* originally was advocated (Dettweiler, 1877) in order to protect the tubercular against the consequences of their dangerous behavioral tendencies—years before the danger of infection had become recognized. For them, the sanitarium not only functioned as a disciplinary measure, but also provided a symbiotic form of *group life* with others who were, quite literally, congenial. Obviously the human milieu of the sanitarium also entailed the danger of becoming seductive, a "Magic Mountain" with its own risks of the emotional frustration that feeds the infectious process.

The isomorphism of life style, Rorschach percepts, and cellular behavior is obvious. As the need for symbiotic human relationships prevails over concern with survival and is reflected in the Rorschach percepts, the genetically tuberculosis-prone subject compensates for the lost human love object by surrendering his/her life to the bond with the bacilli.

In the case of *cancer,* the analogy between personality and cellular behavior is equally evident. As long as the subject succeeds in controlling the *objects of his/her respective dominant organ functions,* the cells of the organ replace themselves according to their specific life spans, although they generally have been exposed to carcinogens or radiation damage for many years or even decades. Only when the subject has experienced the irretrievable loss of the vital object will the cells of the organ begin to grow autistically and form the tumor. This self-created object compensates for the lost environmental object in two respects:

1. the tumor grows in the organ itself and thus cannot be lost;
2. the cells achieve their irresistible expansion because their metabolism has regressed from oxidation to fermentation (Warburg, 1956), from aerobic to anaerobic, the phylogenoetically older life process that entails a life span exceeding that of normal cells.

As in the case of tuberculosis, so in the case of the cancer-prone subject, is the isomorphism of life style, Rorschach percepts, and cellular behavior clear. The need for individual survival prevails over concern with symbiotic human relationships and is reflected in the Rorschach percepts. The subject compensates for the loss of its individualistically controlled object by creating an internal object endowed with vitality superior to his/her own organism. Thus the cancer patient sacrifices his/her life with people on the altar of the idiosyncratic object-relationship.

PLATE IV

Rorschach emphasized that this plate made all interpretations of the whole inkblot difficult. Merei characterized it as evoking "childhood and anxiety."

The psychological demand character of Plate IV is mainly determined by two features:

1. The vertical concentration of dark color suggests the childhood situation of being alone in a dark room.
2. The configuration suggests a single organism or object. It is impossible to see two organisms facing each other, the nearly inevitable percepts of Plates II and III. The suggestion of the darkness is thus enhanced: *being alone and unsupported.*

In the course of growing up probably most people have undergone experiences of feeling lost and helpless, but only a few have been affected so seriously that the suggestions of the fourth inkblot picture cause the so-called "dark shock," an impaired capacity of forming one of the two most common percepts. These percepts are:

1. The outlines of an organism characterized by two big feet, two much smaller arms, and an even less distinct head, suggesting *a human or humanlike creature.* These features are suggestive of the course of events in which the subject has outgrown the total helplessness of the newborn infant: learning to stand, to walk, to use the hands and finally the head, in order to cope with frustrating situations. This basic percept is typical of personalities who are self-reliant when they find themselves deprived of support. The "Charlie Chaplin" figure owes its worldwide popularity to having incorporated these features.
2. The suggestions of four extremities, a big head at the bottom, and a furry texture of the whole add up to the percept of an *animal skin.* This response is typical of individuals who, when feeling unsupported, comfort themselves by reviving infantile experiences of soft and warm contact with the mother. The primary role of the tactile sense in the experience of affectionate support is a biological characteristic of primate

infants. This is evident from the studies of René Spitz on "hospitalism" (1945), from Harry Harlow's experiments (1965, 1970) with cloth surrogate mothers for monkeys, and Tinbergen's observations (1973) of autistic children. The popularity of the blanket of Linus should also be mentioned.

The *first alternative* described above seems to be responsible for the fact that this card has frequently been designated "The Father Card" (Phillips and Smith, 1953), since fathers are expected to stand on their own feet. It is fitting that the self-sufficient patriarchal Swiss should often consider it beautiful, as Rorschach observed. A different image of independence seems to be projected by the French. According to Theodora Abel (1948, 1954), they tend to see foreign invaders in it. The French have certainly remained individualists in the course of their long history, in which they have alternately acted as invaders and been invaded by their neighbors.

THE CANCER CRITERIA

1. The percept of the whole inkblot as an intact organism suggests that the subject feels self-sufficient. The same meaning, in less obvious forms, is implied in the three other criteria.
2. The percept of undomesticated, warmblooded animals (excepting the unspecific "bat" and "bear") suggests a feeling of independence from the conformist expectations of the social environment.
3. Percepts of large size, scariness, or aggression suggest self-assertiveness.
4. Percepts *not* involving hiding, clothing, or a supportive background (cf #4, tuberculosis criteria) suggest that, forced to depend on themselves, cancer patients are not self-protective.

The last-mentioned type of response to Plate IV is particularly noteworthy because it is the opposite of the response to Plate I. Apparently cancer patients avoid self-revelation only when they are confronted with a new situation. Because of their experience of inadequate mothering, they are suspicious of others; but once they have taken the measure of those they are dealing with they treat them with the frankness they consider warranted.

The ongoing controversy about whether cancer patients should be told the truth seems to be due to the fact that *physicians* differ so much in respect of their own attitudes toward death, whereas most of their patients are quite realistic. This means that they outwardly accept the doctor's words and inwardly follow their own life styles. Their percepts of Plate IV illustrate this inner consistency. When they first become suspicious of symptoms (Goldsen et al, 1957; Gold, 1964), they often are reluctant to seek medical help, and allow the dynamics of the pathological process to defeat all therapeutic measures.

Since the time of Galen, physicians have been aware of the depressive quality of cancer patients. Modern physicians are apt to be put off by the evidence of suicidal behavior, because they have put their entire faith in the power of a purely materialistic approach. They have, therefore, been particularly reluctant to engage themselves in the study of the psychosomatic aspects of the cancer, even when psychosomatics became increasingly accepted in the approach to other diseases. Actually it was a clinical psychologist, Lawrence LeShan (LeShan and Worthington, 1956), who first drew renewed attention to the consistent life pattern of cancer patients. Later, the tragic connection between modern medicine and the epidemic increase of cancer-prone personalities became clear with the discovery (Booth, 1969b) that the advances of scientific pediatrics and of bacteriology reduced the mortality of the tuberculosis-prone population at the same rate as that of the increase in cancer mortality.

Fundamentally, this error of medical science can be traced to the profanation of human life implicit in the materialistic development of Western culture, inherent in the Cartesian split of body and soul. Science was carried away by the fantasy that ultimately the organism could be fully understood as a machine and manipulated by physical and chemical methods. At the same time, the Industrial Revolution promised the Millennium as the reward for perfection of materialistic productivity. Together these trends resulted in the facts that the Industrial Revolution sacrificed the natural nursing relationship between mother and child, and that medical science succeeded in raising physically healthy individuals.

Within the last three decades, however, it has become evident that the rise of physical longevity has been achieved at the expense of the psychological health of modern man. Many physicians (Spitz, 1945, 1957, 1965; Newton and Newton, 1967; Booth, 1974a, 1975) have found that natural nursing has a much more complex function than the feeding of babies: that it is the psychobiological foundation for interpersonal relationships of a sexual as well as of a nonsexual nature.

Whereas the social and psychological consequences of the materialistic misunderstanding of man are generally ignored, the cancer epidemic has provided very concrete evidence that the violation of the psychosexual sphere of life has caused a major health problem for the fifth of the population that is genetically tuberculosis prone. Raised according to the standards of physical hygiene, their capacity for psychosexual fulfillment was crippled. Control of individualistic object-relationships can maintain health only up to a point; with the loss of such control, the underlying sexual factor asserts itself in the form of cancerous regression.

The basic function of sex being the guarantee of the survival of the race, the frustrated organ cells regress to the earliest manifestation of the immortality of life. Before there was sexual reproduction, there was reproduction by cell division. As Hayflick demonstrated (1966), cancer cells compensate for the loss of functional differentiation by greater vitality. If they are transplanted into a healthy organism, they outlive the organism of origin and kill their host. In an ironical sense, one may say that modern medicine achieved its goal of conquering death in creating the cancer epidemic: the patient dies, but his cancer cells are potentially immortal. The fundamental principle of sexual propagation remains valid: *the sex cells are immortal, but the individual carriers die.*

In cancer patients, the rationale of sexuality is internalized. Prevented from fulfillment in the form of procreation with the opposite sex, they live healthy lives in the form of intense object relationships mediated by their dominant organ function. Once they have exhausted this possibility, they die in surrendering their vitality to the cancer cells, unless therapy provides new, adequate object relationships. How this is possible will be discussed in the chapter on therapy.

The preceding clinical facts explain the Rorschach findings that indicate that these patients show so much evidence of individualistic strength when they are on their own. Clinically it is well known that usually cancer patients have been healthy, vital personalities before the onset of the disease.

THE TUBERCULOSIS CRITERIA

1. Because of their strong symbiotic needs, the tuberculosis patients frequently reveal in their percepts the very obvious imagery that the mere suggestion of being alone makes them *feel injured.* They therefore see damaged organisms and objects where the cancer patients saw strength. Even the fur

skin, the forerunner of the "security blanket," appears damaged. Nothing but a real dyadic relationship can reassure them.

The majority of the tuberculosis patients manifest their frustrated dependent needs in less self-explanatory percepts.

2. References to animals favor *domesticated animals;* e.g., cowhide. They, like the patients, depend on association with caring human beings.
3. Percepts of details of the inkblot implying small size and weakness express the same meaning as that of criterion #1.
4. The percepts of hiding, clothing, and an imagined support are best understood in context with criterion #3 of Plate I. There, the tuberculosis patients manifested their initial basic trust in the mother relationship in the form of uninhibited self-display. In later life, this basic trust prevented them from using critical judgment in their striving for affection. In Plate IV, the image of a lonely object evokes the crucial trauma of having lost the relationship they had trusted. The type #4 percepts show their attempts at trying to protect themselves as well as their illusionist, "eternally hopeful" reaching out into the void for a new relationship. If frustrated beyond endurance, the relationship will be found with the Koch bacillus.

Keeping in mind that, genetically, both cancer and tuberculosis patients were born with an abnormally strong need for affection, the influence of adequate and inadequate mothering on the form of later somatic disease is most directly illustrated in the contrasting percepts of Plate IV.

In the case of tuberculosis, the affectionate need had been literally nursed by the mother and had made the subject dependent on the continued enjoyment of warm, mutual relationships with others. When they lost this vital satisfaction, they surrendered their bodies to the bacilli that threatened to consume them.

In the case of cancer, the infants were endowed with strong enough vitality to invest their dominant organ function successfully in a limited object-relationship which they could control and which made life worth living. When they lost the vital object-relationship, they compensated for it by creating in the frustrated organ an internalized object that expanded in size until it killed the rest of the organism. As mentioned in the discussion of Plate III, they have identified themselves with the survival needs of the dominant organ. Nature is consistent. Cancer-prone individuals, having survived inadequate mothering thanks to the strength of their survival functions, end their lives by transforming the cells of the dominant organ into cancer cells, which have greater survival capacity than ordinary body cells.

PLATE V

For most subjects (excepting some schizophrenics), the fifth ink-blot is the easiest to perceive as a whole. With the preceding plate, it shares the important feature of suggesting *social isolation,* but it lacks the massing of darkness in the *vertical* dimension of the center that many subjects experience as anxiety-provoking.

The *vertical axis* of this plate is quite insubstantial and the spread of the configuration is *horizontal* and flat, suggesting the popular percepts, "bat" or "butterfly."

Merei (1953) felt that Plate V tested the "relationships to reality" and claimed that, in all cases in which the popular percepts were missed, the reality function was disturbed. "Reality," however, is too wide a concept. A better definition would be "lack of common sense." Such subjects are not satisfied with trivial solutions of the trivial tasks of everyday life, but are driven to express their individualities where most people are content to act "like everybody else." This holds true for the majority of the cancer and tuberculosis patients. Plate V is the only one of the series that most members of these two clinical groups perceive in ways that do not reveal their respective disease liability (see Figure I, p. 244).

The preceding observation explains why the majority of modern physicians has become unaware of the personality types associated with somatic diseases. The growing impersonality of the methods of clinical examination provides, just like Plate V, very little opportunity for observing the personality of the patient. Whereas formerly the physician had to rely on the personal history, subjective symptoms, and his own sensory examination of the body, in modern times diagnosis and therapy are derived from x-rays and instrument readings. Concentration on the technological approach leaves hardly any time for attention to the person who creates the physical, electrical, and chemical data.

The subjects who do produce disease-specific percepts of Plate V express the same psychological attitudes that were discussed in the context of Plate IV. Cancer patients respond to the experience of isolation with a display of their strong survival instinct, whereas the tuberculosis patients are reminded that they can satisfy their symbiotic need only by surrendering to the bacillus.

PLATE VI

Rorschach observed that this card is experienced as most difficult to interpret, but he gave no explanation. There is no evidence that he had planned the configuration for the purpose of testing sexual behavior; but it is a fact that the two most conspicuous axial areas contain symbolizations of a phallus on top of a vulva. Because of the multiple-choice structure of all the inkblots, the symbolization of genital organs is not noticed by most subjects, for the general appearance of the inkblot is weighted in favor of non-genital percepts. Only subjects who find it difficult to integrate their sexual impulses with their personal relationships perceive isolated genital organs. Many others, however, unconsciously give evidence of being influenced by the genital features. In some cases this is suggested by the wording of their responses, in others by association with the percepts, sometimes by their handling of the card—they may turn it upside down, or cover part of it with their hand, or stroke the "furry skin."

The combination of the suggestion of female genitals with the suggestion of a fur skin is one of the most striking manifestations of Rorschach's intuitive understanding of psychodynamics. This "inkblot" anticipated Harlow's (1965) monkey experiments with "cloth mother surrogates," which clarified the development of affectionate behavior in primates. Specifically, Harlow proved that both sexes develop the capacity for sexual intercourse only if the animals have experienced, as infants, interaction with the furry body of the mother or, in the case of dummy-raised infants, with the bodies of playmates.

The biological link between "soft object," affection, and development of coital competence in primates apparently is rooted in the satisfaction of the infantile "clinging reflex" by a living mother (Hermann, 1936). If the biological association between the soft object and the maternal body is artificially frustrated the infants of monkeys and of modern mothers spontaneously cling to inanimate soft objects such as their crib blankets as if they represented security—hence the "security blanket" of the popular comic strip character Linus in "Peanuts." The observation of this behavior led Harlow to the creation of his "cloth surrogate mother" and modern mothers to the creation of rag dolls and buying of Teddy bears. In both species, the result is the same: the infants become adults who respond to the bodies of their mates with instinctual sexual

behavior as if they were inanimate. The capacity for mutual co-
ordination of their sexual reflexes did not develop. Although human
adults intellectually know what is required, they generally become com-
petent only by the Masters and Johnson technique (1970), which is
based on developing the capacity for pleasurable body contact prior to
any genital activity.

In addition to the biological aspects of the sexual sphere of existence,
just discussed, the subject's responses to Plate VI are apt to reflect
social problems between the sexes. The separation of the inkblot into
two contiguous, but very dissimilar, subdivisions makes it very difficult
to perceive the whole inkblot as a unit. This device effectively symbolizes
the social problem of the coexistence of the two sexes. We know from
anthropology that mankind has developed an amazing number of social
solutions of the biological problem that, in fulfilling their procreative
functions, both sexes partly need each other, partly need autonomy.
The problem is certainly not manmade, since botany and zoology provide
far greater varieties of solutions.

THE CANCER CRITERIA

1. Cancer patients tend to experience the sensuous and seductive
   aspects of sex as a threat to their individualistic form of
   existence, because of an infantile experience of inadequate
   mothering. They therefore do not respond to the rather
   obvious "fur skin," or they see it in an artificially reduced
   form.
2. The need for autonomy is also expressed in the fact that
   cancer patients tend to ignore the physical fusion of the
   "male" and "female" areas of the inkblot. Sexual and non-
   sexual percepts of the two areas ignore their spatial relationship.
3. Self-sufficiency appears also in the fact that even those who
   do perceive the "fur skin" do not manifest a tendency to
   reach beyond the boundaries of the given area, a trait already
   encountered in Plate IV, #4, that also often elicits percepts
   of furriness.

All the criteria suggest that cancer patients tend to assert their
individualism in their sexual behavior, although, at least on the
unconscious level, most of them have proven capable of the eminently
symbiotic acts of begetting progeny, and many have consciously pursued sexual satisfaction, often with great intensity, like Harlow's

"motherless monkeys." The sexual individualism of cancer patients manifests itself, not so much in their physical activities, but very strongly in the ways in which they experience them as physical needs that conflict with their striving for "object control." This is most evident in patients whose cancers are localized in their sexual organs (cf. Section B of this chapter.).

The "cancer view" of sexuality has been incorporated and masterfully analyzed in Freud's psychological research, which began to focus on sex 30 years prior to his cancer of the jaw. His theory and his own case fully illustrate that the cancer-prone personality exists prior to the disease. Freud soon became convinced that the biological interdependence of male and female involves degradation (1908). Castration fear and penis envy seemed inevitable to him; he considered them the "organic rock bottom" that ultimately limits the therapeutic possibilities of psychoanalysis. Thus, he asserted at the end of his life that the "repudiation of femininity must surely be a biological fact, part of the great riddle of sex" (1937).

THE TUBERCULOSIS CRITERIA

1. The percept of the "fur skin" suggests that tuberculosis patients have started life with an adequate infantile experience of mothering, which made it possible for them to develop the capacity for mature heterosexual relationships.
2. Since physiological heterosexuality leads to intimate fusion in spite of the physical differences of the sexes and the different individualities of the mates, the tuberculosis patients tend to *perceive the spatial contact between the "male" and the "female" parts of the inkblot in terms of a functional interrelationship,* mostly without awareness of sexual implications.
3. Percepts of the "fur skin" as being in contact with an imagined environment express (cf. Plate IV, #3) that the need for symbiotic contact disposes these subjects toward imaginary wish fulfillments.

The percepts of Plate VI prevailing among cancer patients on the one hand and tuberculosis patients on the other hand, lead to the conclusion that the two clinical groups differ significantly in respect of their basic sexual attitudes (cf. Chapter VIII). In describing these divergencies no consideration has been given to observations of individual cases in which neurotic and/or psychotic distortions are apt to disguise the underlying constitutional tendencies. Cancer patients may have been compulsive and jealous lovers, tuberculosis patients may have been sexually inhibited and expressed their genital needs in the form of neurotic symptom formations. Such cases are not within the scope of this research, based as it is on the Rorschach records of patients, most of whom I never saw. One clinical example of neurotic distortion, however, can be given for the psychodynamics behind such responses to Plate VI.

"A glass plunger in a vagina," if scored mechanically, would fall under the second type of tuberculosis response, but closer psychological consideration suggests the implication that a contraceptive device defends the individual against commitment to a sexual relationship. In this case of lung cancer, an inquiry into the biographical facts was possible. This was a professional woman who had separated her genital activities from the rest of her life. She jealously guarded her autonomy, both in relation to the men who provided intense, though rarely orgastic, sexual satisfaction, and to those with whom she maintained an intellectual dialogue on a very high level.

PLATE VII

Rorschach pointed out that the most important feature of this card is the large expanse of white space that separates the two lateral expanses of the inkblot. The resulting configuration makes it valuable as a test of the reaction to a situation the subject cannot control. The main features are:

1. The broad expanse of white space in the center, and the suggestion of a split of the blot at the bottom, make it impossible to form a satisfactory percept of one organism as center of the field. Such percepts are made easy in Plate IV and V, and possibly in Plate I. Subjects anxious to dominate situations find the central emptiness very frustrating, and they try to cope with the disturbing gestalt by turning the card upside down. This maneuver represents a two-fold escape from the reality demand:

    a) top and bottom of the real world cannot be reversed arbitrarily;

    b) the turning of the card facilitates percepts of the white space as a solid object and of the disturbing lateral inkblots as mere background. The content of the white-space interpretations often expresses power fantasies—

heads of Napoleon, George Washington, the Sphinx, the tip of an arrow or of a penis.

Subjects made insecure by the structure of Plate VII thus compensate their anxieties by perceiving in the empty space images of power, and ignoring the inkblot itself.

2. The two lateral areas of the inkblot make it easy to perceive them as two people or animals. This basic feature is the same as in Plates II and III, but there is one important difference: Several special features of Plate VII suggest that the equality of the two symmetrical figures is threatened. Not only do they look off balance, but also the seesaw shape of the bottom area implies an unstable level of dominance between them. At the same time, their being topped by headgear expresses a striving for social superiority. The whole configuration makes it difficult to perceive for subjects who feel *insecure in interpersonal relationships* in which they are not supported by either strong emotions (Plate II) or social conventions (Plate III). These subjects either fail to recognize the human features of the lateral areas or else attribute to them hostile affects.

Because Plate VII frequently elicits associations with childhood experiences, many Rorschach psychologists have interpreted it as the "mother card," without sound perceptanalytic justification (Piotrowski, 1957). Their superficial generalization, however, points up a very unfortunate truth: many modern subjects do *associate their experience of the mother with insecure interpersonal relationships.* This observation contradicts the traditional assumption that the instinctual bond between mother and child makes this relationship the most secure one. This assumption, however, was generally justified only as long as the relationship between mothers and children was securely founded on the mutual biological satisfaction of breast feeding, which maintained a dyadic relationship during the first year of extrauterine existence (Newton and Newton, 1967). In the centuries of high infant mortality, only those women became mothers who had been successfully nursed and were therefore capable of transmitting their mothering instincts to their daughters, except for the small minority of upper-class women who surrendered their babies to wet nurses. The latter often were not very motherly, and contributed to the frequency of "degeneracy" among the children of upper-class parents (Chapter VII, B will discuss this point).

Infant care *changed radically in the 19th century.* Then, for the first time in the history of the human race, a constantly increasing proportion of children reached maturity without having experienced an adequate dyadic mother relationship. The Industrial Revolution initiated the change by making breast feeding economically unbearable for proletarian mothers, even though hand feeding resulted in particularly high infant mortality. Gradually, however, the invention of the rubber nipple and the progress of scientific medicine made the chances of physical survival equal for bottle-fed and breast-fed infants. Science having become the religion of the modern age, more and more mothers and physicians turned to artificial feeding. This trend has continued, although in 1945—the centenary of the rubber nipple—René Spitz (1965) discovered that bottle feeding entailed grave risks for the physical and social health of the infants because it easily involved frustration of their dyadic needs.

Although the scientific soundness of Spitz's research has not been faulted, only few physicians and educated women have heeded his warnings. Neither have they paid attention to the fact that epidemic tuberculosis began to recede in the middle of the 19th century at the same rate at which the incidence of cancer grew to its present epidemic dimension, and that this transformation coincided with the growing number of artificially fed individuals reaching cancer age (Booth, 1969b). The conclusion from the epidemiological facts should have been obvious for the past 70 years, that cancer is the result of the impact of modern nursing practices on genetically tuberculosis-prone infants. But the fact is so unpleasant to face, that I realized only after several years that my Rorschach data (1964b) linked the findings of Spitz with those of Thomas Cherry (1924, 1925) and of other statisticians. Since 1967, I have presented the preceding observations at six international medical meetings devoted to the cancer problem, without encountering criticism in the ensuing discussions, or from the editors who published my papers. Nevertheless, so far nobody seems to have made use of this work. The implication of an iatrogenic factor in the cancer epidemic is unpalatable indeed.

THE CANCER CRITERIA

1. The individualistic world view of cancer-prone subjects frequently prevents them from perceiving the two popular lateral figures, but conditions them to perceive single objects that either are coextensive with the whole inkblot or at least are co-axial with the axis of symmetry. Significantly, this perceptual behavior implies that these subjects find it easier

to relate to inanimate objects than to involve themselves in human relationships on the level of equality.

The trend toward percepts of inanimate objects has a psychological meaning that is best explained by Martin Buber's (1937) concept of "I - It" relationships. The other person is experienced as separate, excluded from the mutuality described as "I - Thou" relationship. Cancer-prone subjects tend to deal with their fellow human beings unilaterally, although frequently in a spirit of kindness and generosity. The underlying "I -It" is apt to create problems with persons who are sensitive in this respect.

The ultimate biological consequence of the trend just described is represented by the role of carcinogens in the disease. Carcinogens are always inanimate. Even the frequently suspected viruses cannot multiply except as parts of living cells. Normal body cells usually have not been in contact with carcinogens for many years or decades prior to the disease. Cancer cells develop and multiply only in the cancer-prone person who undergoes the experience of having forever lost control over his/her conscious vital object, which may be a person, a collective situation, or a personal project. In this predicament, such a person regresses to making a carcinogen the object of last resort. Together, person and carcinogen create the tumor, the unconscious substitute of the lost conscious object.

A dramatic historical example of the carcinogenic situation, the case of the late Senator Taft, was described in the discussion of Plate III. The psychobiological specificity of the cancer reaction to loss of power is highlighted by the contrasting history of Winston Churchill, whose death from cardiovascular disease made him representative of this personality type. He only lived by his faith that he was right, and thus he survived several crushing political defeats after he had reached cancer age. The resulting free time he used for historical writings. Thus he found satisfaction as observer of world events when politics prevented him from being a leader.

2. The tendency to perceive the whole inkblot as a group of six objects of the same kind is a specific expression of the self-contained attitude prevailing in the cancer group. This type of percept presupposes that the subject is not very interested in the rather pronounced differences between the shapes of the three pairs of major details.

The psychological implication of these percepts is the same as that of the type #1, just discussed: the need for self-sufficient existence. But they also reveal another aspect of the cancer personality which, at first sight, seems contradictory: the cancer-prone need to be part of a group that tolerates their autonomy. In other words, the genetic need for symbiotic existence has survived, although on a biologically regressive level. E. Forgue pointed out (1931) that cancer patients should not be isolated after surgery. H.B. Andervont (1944) found that mice in crowded cages did not develop cancer, even if sexual activity were excluded. J.V. Fiddian (1930) drew attention to the similarity between the behavior of cancer cells and the gregariousness of amoebae. And Hayflick (1966) discovered that the cells of Carrel tissue cultures owed their immortality to cancerous transformation.

The congruity between the self-contained behavior of cancer patients and their percepts of Plate VII is well illustrated by the example of a successfully operated lung cancer patient. He had been a New York taxi driver for 23 years and was particularly proud of the fact that his cab had never been scratched in traffic. "I never got nervous, only my passengers got nervous because I would rather arrive on the following day than take any risks." He gave two quite original responses to Plate VII that reflect his attitude toward interpersonal relationships:

> two little *puppets* on a see-saw;
> modern painting of two elephants *back to back*,
>   standing up on their hind legs with raised trunks!

THE TUBERCULOSIS CRITERIA

1. The powerful symbiotic need of these patients favors the popular percept of two human beings facing each other.
2. The awareness of the risky interpersonal relationship suggested by Plate VII is reflected in nearly half of the tuberculosis patients in percepts implying an unstable situation, whereas not one of my 125 cancer records showed such percepts.

The conclusion is drawn that tuberculosis patients prefer self-destructive interpersonal relationships to none at all. They therefore tolerate awareness of the risks inherent in their way of living. There is only one exception: 23 percent of the patients with unfavorable prognosis were incapable of forming any percept of Plate VII. In fatal cases, apparently the image of unstable human relationships has a shock effect. They no longer cope with their frustrated needs for symbiotic fulfillment in symbiosis with the mycobacterium tuberculosis.

The structure of Plate VII demands acceptance of an unstable and uncontrollable interpersonal relationship. Cancer patients frequently avoid this by finding satisfaction in dealing with inanimate objects.

Biologically, this takes the form of reaction with carcinogens.

PLATE VIII

Rorschach saw the essential characteristics of this plate in the use of four different colors, the harmony of colors and forms, the easy interpretation of the separate colored areas, and the production of "color shock" in neurotics.

Rorschach's terse statement does not reveal whether he was conscious that he had structured the inkblot into a symbol of the *harmonious aspect of nature*. This effect is achieved by the subtle use of forms and colors *in the axial area* of the blot.

1. The *forms* of the colored areas make it impossible for most subjects to perceive them as organisms [with which] they can empathize, but they nevertheless convey a feeling of naturalness. This graphic fact seems to be symbolic of the biological existence of man, which is made possible by infinitely complex and mostly unknown structures and processes. We take them for granted, like the ground on which we stand.

2. The *colors* of the axial area are arranged in a striking order: the colors are warm at the bottom, cool in the middle, and cold gray at the top. This constellation corresponds to two levels of the evolution of human life:

   a) The *evolution of our planet* as a fiery ball is still present as its hot core; the cooling of the crust allowed the formation of oceans, the breeding ground of life. The blueish-green often is perceived as the sea, and reminds the biologist of the primal photosynthetic micro-organisms that created the oxygen of our atmosphere. The mountains rise above the range of life and point up into the cosmic space in which the earth originated. All over the world one finds evidence that archaic man perceived mountains as the seats of gods, of superhuman creative powers.

   b) The *evolution of man* is symbolized by the polarity of the red bottom and the gray top. Animal warmth—the circulation of blood—is the basis of all organ functions in differentiated creatures, and the outreaching "gray matter" at the top enables man to control his own body and to interact with his environment.

The preceding interpretation of the axial areas as representing the unconscious core of existence is in keeping with the placement of the two vertebrate creatures in the periphery of the inkblot. Their position and the fragmentation of the "ground" under their feet represent the precarious nature of individual existence in the depersonalized natural environment and the need for individual action in order to avoid falling off into space. Many subjects avoid facing this disturbing image by turning the plate sideways. This maneuver makes "the animal" stand on top of a mountain and suggests the human fantasy of man as the conqueror of nature. But even this manipulation does not dispose of the fact that the animal's stance remains insecure, since one leg is suspended over a lot of empty space.

The total effect of the inkblot picture adds up to the image of the mysterious order of the natural world, in which individuals, however, exist on the strength of their own efforts.

THE CANCER CRITERIA

1. Cancer patients tend to perceive anatomical or pathological structures in the axial area because the latter frustrates their need to see every situation as individually controlled. The inkblot is dominated by a mountainlike form, and only unusually imaginative subjects are capable of seeing it as a live organism. The expanse of four colors along the axis invites emotional arousal and involvement, a feature that easily induces avoidance reactions in cancer-prone subjects (cf. Plate III, #3), whose primary need is autonomy. The perception of dead or sick objects in the center is in keeping with the fate of cancer patients: When the function that has dominated his/her life has become irretrievably frustrated, its executive organ asserts its power through the regression of its cells to the undifferentiated vitality of primordial life, killing the less-valued remainder of the organism.

2. The isolation of the lateral "animals" satisfies the autonomous needs of cancer patients so much that they tend to ignore the unnatural color and the precarious stance and to perceive the creatures in free action. The determination to persevere in defiance of a frustrating environment characterizes the lives of cancer patients. Ever since the first months of life, their survival instincts, their "ego," have compensated for the life-threatening experience of inadequate mothering. As pointed out above (Plate IV, #4), this vital power of perseverance

involves the subjects' reluctance to pay attention to symptoms of beginning disease.

3. The prevailing decisiveness of their percepts is particularly striking in view of the fact that the visual data of all the major areas is ambiguous. Even the "animals" are suggestive of practically any four-legged vertebrate. If the area is just called "an animal," the question, "Which kind?" generally elicits a more specific percept that defines a significant self-identification.

The percepts of the solitary active animal are symbolic of the behavior of cancer tissue, which continues to move ahead on the strength of regression to autonomous anaerobic metabolism.

THE TUBERCULOSIS CRITERIA

1. The axial areas are easily perceived as natural objects because the adequate dyadic mother relationship of tuberculosis patients is easily extended to a dyadic experience of "Mother Nature" in all its manifestations.

2. The symbiotic need of tuberculosis patients makes them *anxious for physical contact,* not only with other human beings, but also with all of nature. They therefore are sensitive to the fact that the "animal" is only to a very limited extent in contact with the ground on which it moves. This awareness leads to percepts of the animal either as motionless or as endangered, because the subjects' health depends on an adequately supportive environment. The consequence has therefore often been a fluctuation between spurts of environment-induced activity alternating with a passive, vegetative existence. In *The Magic Mountain,* Thomas Mann created a classical evocation of this precarious way of life.

3. Tuberculosis patients often feel insecure about their percepts because they are so dependent on environmental support. This dependent need is definitely frustrated by the structure of Plate VIII. The most congenial support obviously would be an image of contact with one's own kind; but the two symmetrical animals are separated by the mountainous area that blocks awareness of each other, in contrast to the symmetrical creatures in Plates I-III and VII. The only immediately available supports are the crags and crannies

under their feet. The main body of the inkblot offers opportunity for many percepts that are tentative rather than reassuring, as unstable as the life histories of these patients.

Plate VIII tests the subject's perception of his/her individual existence in a life situation that emphasizes the rational and emotionally balanced features of the natural environment.

Cancer patients feel secure under these circumstances because their deprived infancy has prepared them to make the most of the opportunities offered by reality. This inner security is maintained even when its external support is lost. In this case, *autonomy* becomes the ultimate expression of personality. Its assertion is more highly valued than survival, as this single-minded pursuit often entails delay or even total rejection of medical intervention.

Tuberculosis patients do not feel secure, because the dyadic experience of infancy has made them inordinately dependent on continued sharing of affectionate mutual relationships. All reality situations that do not offer adequate satisfaction of this need therefore involve the danger of seeking unconscious fulfillment in symbiosis with the mycobacterium tuberculosis.

PLATE IX

Rorschach planned this inkblot as a contrast to the preceding one by making it disharmonious in colors and forms, by combining in one plate features that individually had constituted specific problems in preceding plates, and by adding some further difficulties.

1. As in Plate II, differently colored areas overlap and remind the subject that our emotions cannot be clearly defined or separated.

2. As in Plate VII, a central space separates the two top areas and suggests a situation that makes impossible the percept of a centrally controlled gestalt. Once more, competition for dominance is suggested by the "headgear" motif, and once more the two opposing figures are in a state of poor equilibrium, falling backwards. These anxiety-provoking features are further enhanced by the thin lines connecting the two figures and discouraging the implication of Plate VII, that the competitors could get away from each other.

3. Whereas in the preceding Plates II, III, and VIII, colored areas were always used in juxtaposition with achromatic areas, providing an *escape from emotional stimuli into the*

sphere of rationality, Plate IX is fully colored.

4. The ninth plate demands acceptance of considerably greater expressionistic distortions than any of the other plates do in order to discover representational human and animal forms. The subject can find meaning only by imaginatively transcending the contours of the actual physical areas.

5. This plate more than any other except Plate VI suggests a *vertical polarity* in addition to the polarity between the symmetrical side figures. A contrast between "down to earth" and "up to heaven" is suggested by the following features:

   a) the forms are solid and rounded at the bottom, thin and pointed at the top;

   b) the colors are strong at the bottom and get weaker toward the top. In particular, the central space is given a blueish tinge in contrast to the purple bottom area, suggesting the contrast between the ethereal and the material spheres of life. The plate is often interpreted as "hell, earth, and heaven," or "four apples on the ground" and "flames on top." Responses to the vertical structure of this card often indicate how the individual tries to solve his relationship with reality, on a materialistic or on a transcendental level.

Summing up the complex demands of Plate IX, one may say that it evokes in concentrated form the inescapable complexities of *individual existence.* They seem to defy a satisfactory solution on the levels of physical reality and of pure intellect. Thus the reaction to this card tests specifically the strength of the ego in facing the irrationalities of life. This conclusion agrees with Merei's, that it tests the "capacity for work and achievement;" I would add: "under favorable conditions."

THE CANCER CRITERIA

The constitutional vitality of cancer patients is manifest in the fact that only eight percent of them were so dismayed by the massed difficulties of Plate IX that they completely failed to form any percept. The typical percepts of the others suggest:

1. Under the impact of an inescapable existential crisis their physiological functions disintegrate even more drastically than when they are confronted with the mere demand for emotional responsiveness (see Plate VIII, #1).

2. They tend to ignore the suggestion of interpersonal engage-

ment. Even when they are in serious trouble, they do not avail themselves of human support on a level of equality. They never overcome the initial despair about human relationships that resulted from the experience of inadequate mothering.

3. The low frequency of kinesthetic percepts of human and of animal forms highlights the meaning of criterion #2: The initiative of cancer patients faced with vital risks is paralyzed by situations in which they are confronted with equals. The kinesthetic responses to Plate VIII show that they are acting purposefully when equals are screened out and they feel in control. It is obvious that, as they grow older, this condition of health becomes more and more difficult to maintain because vitality declines and social problems multiply for those who have been constitutionally incapable of developing relationships based on mutual affection.

There is only one group of cancers that deviates from the general tendency to avoid interpersonal involvement even under great stress: the patients whose tumors were localized in genital organs. Since they perceived the preceding eight plates like other cancer patients, their percepts of Plates IX and X will be discussed separately in the following Section B (p. 116).

THE TUBERCULOSIS CRITERIA

The response of tuberculosis patients to the difficulties symbolized in Plate IX is affected in a general way by their clinical condition. Of the group with an unfavorable prognosis, 27 percent failed to form any percept, whereas only 2.4 percent failed in the group that had a good prognosis. Apparently only when the vitality of tuberculosis patients is severely depleted do they tend to give up conscious interaction with the environment. Otherwise they try to maintain object relationship in the following forms:

1. Even under great stress, tuberculosis patients maintain their symbiotic attitude. Thus they keep aware of the ongoing life in their environment and the opportunities for interaction, whereas cancer patients abandon symbiotic life in favor of autistic cell proliferation.

2. Percepts of the spiky orange connections between the two top figures as aggressive suggest that their need for interpersonal involvement is so strong that they would rather

enact it aggressively than give up. This is very noteworthy because the whole genetic group is characterized by a low level of aggressive tendencies.

3. The kinesthetic percepts of human and of animal forms suggest that even very trying situations do not easily discourage their needs for symbiotic interaction, although it may regress to the unconscious level of the infectious process. Their "eternal hopefulness" keeps them alerted to possibilities of returning to the more satisfactory level of congenial human relationships, which accounts for the frequency of remissions. Obviously, this readiness for hope can also be completely unrealistic and lead to self-destructive behavior. Two patients perceived in Plate IX the story of Icarus: the orange top as the youth flying toward the sun, defying his father's warning that the wax that fastened the feathers to his artificial wings would melt; and the red bottom area as his smashed body on the ground.

The symbolization of a very difficult life situation in Plate IX elicits contrasting perceptual tendencies that suggest the following interpretations:

Cancer patients despair when they find no possibility of maintaining control. They become passive and regress from physiological aerobic life to anaerobic metabolism in the organ of the frustrated function.

Tuberculosis patients continue to maintain their symbiotic form of existence and keep trying to find fulfillment in human relationships and, in case of failure, regress to the destructive symbiosis with the aerobic bacilli.

PLATE X

Rorschach had three points in mind when he constructed this card: "Multi-colored. Disjointed blots. Near impossibility of a response to the whole." A more detailed analysis of the perceptual conditions, in the light of clinical experience, is in order:

1. "Multi-colored": This condition appeared in the two preceding plates, but only in this one are all major chromatic and achromatic colors united in one plate. Thus a maximum opportunity of choice is provided for expression of individual color affinities. The possibilities of choice are further enhanced by the fact that the six different colors appear in 14 different shapes. Thus the whole arrangement represents

symbolically the many emotional and rational *possibilities of life* from which the individual makes his idiosyncratic choices.

2. "Disjointed blots": This impression is favored by the different coloring of the details; but closer attention to the outlines reveals that only two of the 18 distinctly colored areas are completely separated from the 16 tenuously interconnected ones. Awareness of this physical continuum manifests a strong need for physical coherence with the environment; unawareness of the interconnections reflects tolerance of free coexistence with heterogeneous individualities.

3. "Near impossibility of a response to the whole": The nine preceding plates have as a common characteristic a certain simplicity of form and of color arrangement, suggesting that interpretation as one whole picture is demanded and possible. The last card faces such an intention on the part of the subject with an infinitely more complex task. It is significant that the most satisfactory interpretations as a whole are nature scenes. The untold varieties of the inanimate and animate forms of nature often appear to the naive observer to be as grotesquely dissimilar and unconnected as the "disjointed blots" Rorschach intended for the final plate. Since ecology has been taking a closer look at the web of life, it has become increasingly evident that there are many invisible threads that hold its creatures together, very much like the usually overlooked extensions of the "disjointed blots."

The preceding observations lead to the interpretation that Rorschach created a symbol of man's experience of the world: a structured whole of which he can understand and handle only fragments. The specific qualities of these fragments are perceived according to the subject's constitution and experiences, and form the basis of his *attitude toward the future.* Manifestations of this attitude are frequently brought out by the last inkblot because it offers a wide, relatively unstructured variety of perceptual choices, after the inkblots that went before have forced the subject to focus his attention on nine crucial existential situations beginning with infancy. Thus, perceptual decisions are made in the light of a concentrated review of past experiences.

The symbolic significance of the last plate is highlighted by a detail that, for three decades, eluded the attention of countless psychiatrists and psychologists: The various blots constitute a basic gestalt that builds itself up from a broad and intensely colored foundation to a narrow, gray top formed by two straight parallel lines; this culminating part is cut off near the upper margin of the card by a sharp line, as if a knife had been used. The resulting form is radically different from the forms in which the preceding inkblots culminate, all being rounded or pointed like forms in nature. This configuration is an apt symbol of the course of life toward death: Starting on the level of down-to-earth instinctual and emotional dyadic existence, it rises through a sphere of many possibilities, then it gradually narrows down to fewer and fewer choices until it ends altogether.

In keeping with the general human tendency to avoid thoughts about one's own death, the vast majority of viewers has ignored the "cut"; in fact, many even ignore the whole gray top. Even Henri Ellenberger (1958) realized only after he had published his biography of Rorschach (1954), in a sudden flash of intuition, while lecturing, that the cut was precognitive of the tragic end of Rorschach's own life: he died at the age of 37 from a ruptured appendix, less than a year after he had published his outstanding and belatedly appreciated "Psychodiagnostics" (1921).

The final inkblot, even more than the preceding ones, raises the question of how much it is the result of unconscious intuition, and how much a conscious artistic design. Rorschach certainly knew Greek mythology, the story of the three Fates who gather disjointed fibers, spin them into the threads of individual lives, and finally cut them; but we will never know what he thought when he gathered disjointed inkblots into a gestalt that ends in the form of a gray thread cut at the end. This interpretation of the plate is supported by the fact that the central white space twice suggests the shape of an arrowhead, symbol of the flight of time. The shape is clear at the bottom between the green areas and a bit more vague between the pink details.

The uncanny precognitive feature of Rorschach's design of this plate is more than a coincidence. I have records of three patients who were in excellent physical health when they consulted me for psychological problems. After they had developed fatal diseases many years later, I discovered that certain of their Rorschach percepts contained unusual imagery which anticipated the very unusual circumstances of their deaths.

Similar conclusions about Plate X have been reached by other observers. Hector Ritey (1941), for instance, called it, "The Future... everything is possible." Merei (1953) conceptualized it in Lewinian terms as: "The organism-environment field [der Lebensraum]...the sum total of potential events...Practical people...give popular responses and like this card...those who dislike it have turned away from the world. In states of depression and blocking the organism-environment field is contracted. People who fear life express this in the contents of their responses."

The following discussion will show that cancer and tuberculosis patients also express their attitudes toward death in their percepts of Plate X.

THE CANCER CRITERIA

1. The tendency of cancer patients to perceive the whole inkblot as one integrated picture expresses their lifelong need for controlling the objects of their dominant function. When realistic losses rob them of this conscious satisfaction, the uncontrollable growth of the frustrated cells becomes the expression of this vital need and potentially survives the rest of the organism. Unconsciously the identification of the patient with his/her dominant function persists to the end. Just as they tend to deny the need for medical intervention in the beginning, they stoically accept the final stage of the disease. In the words of a great oncologist: "Escape from restraint is fundamental to neoplasia. Physiological isolation, with its many causes, may well be the most important single factor predisposing to the reassertion of that life force to which, in certain circumstances, we give the name of cancer." (Smithers, 1964)

2. The tendency to ignore differentiating forms and colors of the disjointed inkblots in order to form more inclusive perceptual units expresses the same need as criterion #1: The subjects are inclined to ignore the basic fact that life manifests itself in a profusion of heterogeneous, but mutually interacting, organisms. Having been denied, as infants, adequate participation in a dyadic relationship with their mothers, they find it more difficult than tuberculosis patients do to accept the heterogeneous personalities of others. They have survived on the strength of their oral and anal instincts which incorporate, assimilate, and dispose of heterogeneous organisms, just as the cancer grows at the expense of less valued organs. Cancer patients disregard the individualities of others, a behavior that has been misinterpreted as evidence of repressed hostility. This makes as little sense as calling

eating a hostile act. When not hungry, beasts of prey ignore
the animals on which they feed.

3. The lack of interest in the gray area at the top of the total
gestalt is in keeping with the lack of interest in the future
that is so often evident in cancer patients. Thus, they ignore
the highest part of the inkblot, to which the two "arrows of
time" point.

Biologically, the future of life is represented by the genital function.
Throughout many stages of evolution, sex has ruled the lives of male
and female individuals by "blind instinct," forcing them to copulate
and, often, to make elaborate provisions for the future of progeny they
never would meet; e.g., certain wasps paralyze caterpillars, deposit their
eggs in them, and then bury them, thus providing fresh meat for the
larvae when they come out of the eggs. On the higher levels of evolution,
conscious parental behavior developed, expressed in the form of risking
one's own life in defense of the young. "Women and children first" is
still the moral rule in catastrophic situations. Although the future
orientation of biological evolution is thus preserved in our cultural
tradition, it has been seriously weakened in the biological orientation of
a growing number of modern individuals.

In connection with Plates IV and VI, I discussed the way cancer-
prone individuals have become the principal victims of the shift from
breast feeding to bottle feeding. As Niles and Michael Newton pointed
out (1967): "The survival of the human race, long before the concept
of 'duty' evolved, depended upon the two voluntary acts of reproduction—coitus and breast feeding. These had to be sufficiently pleasurable
to ensure their frequent occurrence." They *used* to be pleasurable
because they satisfied two phases of the unitary instinctual organization
on which mammalian reproduction is based: the nursing reaction between
mother and infant prepares the infants of both sexes for future coital
interaction and the production of new infants. In other words, from
generation to generation each behavioral phase conditions the organism
for the following behavioral phase in the service of the preservation of
the species.

In this future-oriented sequence, the *alimentary* function of nursing
is only a secondary implement of procreation, whereas, to the age of
materialistic individualism, babies were considered able to survive and
grow like plants as long as they were fed. Thus, medicine blindly broke
the physiological link between the infant and the future of the human
race by supporting only the instincts of self-preservation. Although the
clinical observations of Spitz (1965), the experiments of Harlow (1965),

and the spreading of sexual incompetence (Masters and Johnson, 1970) have provided ample authoritative warnings that depersonalized nursing interferes with the development of psychosexual maturity, only a statistically insignificant number of educated women and physicians have been moved to take responsible action. Admittedly, the task is difficult; but tackling it seems to be more important for dealing with the cancer epidemic than the current pursuit of carcinogenic substances in our physical environment. *Effective prophylasix will have to begin at birth,* although such a program involves serious problems.[7]

The cancer patients' low concern with the future probably has no major clinical effect on their prognosis. Only five percent failed to form any percepts of Plate X. The great vitality which, in infancy, allowed them to survive the frustration of their dyadic needs stays with them and keeps them going in spite of the disease, on the strength of their survival instincts. This staying power explains how quite a few of them who had been declared incurable have achieved spontaneous regression when an auspicious change in their situation helped them to overcome their carcinogenic despair (Booth, 1973).

The low rate of failures in Plate X is noteworthy in view of my group of hypertensive patients. Although all of these were fairly healthy, 12 percent of them failed to make any response to this plate. Apparently their constitutional dependency on social conformity makes them less capable of making decisions concerning their future than is the case for the individualistic cancer patients.

THE TUBERCULOSIS CRITERIA

1. Tuberculosis patients are less motivated to seek control of their objects because they started life in a trusting relationship with their mothers, the only object of which most infants are aware during the first months of life. Tuberculosis patients, therefore, tolerate more easily than cancer patients the variety of separate heterogeneous details and easily ignore those that do not fit into their symbiotic life experience. Only in the group with a bad prognosis, 20 percent failed to form any percepts, in keeping with their unconscious surrender to the infectious disease.

2. The "basic trust" (Erikson, 1963) of tuberculosis patients is particularly evident in their percepts of disintegration in this last plate. The structure of the inkblot systematically frustrates their dominant need for symbiotic experience of life. Although

there are nine pairs of symmetrical forms, they are all separated (in contrast to Plates I-IV, VII, and IX), the five lateral blots by the gray and pink areas. The four close to each other are separated by four singular axial blots that invite independent, self-contained percepts: The light gray, the orange, blue, and green. The effect is somewhat analogous to that of Plate VIII, in which the two symmetrical animals are separated by the "mountainous" rise between them and frustrated symbiotic needs.

The cumulative imagery of frustrated mutuality creates anxiety, but the percepts also confirm the abiding effect of the infantile dyadic experience. Tuberculosis patients accept experiences of being separated from objects of their symbiotic needs without being discouraged from continued participation in life as long as they find opportunity for establishing new congenial relationships. Their tendency to subdivide solid inkblots into percepts of interrelated smaller percepts appears to be analogous to the infectious process in which a body organ becomes the locale of interaction between its own cells and the bacilli. The "eternal hopefulness" of the patients, in spite of the ravages of the disease, sometimes to the very end, is based on their constitutional capacity for enjoying symbiotic relationships, even though they be on the limited scale of invalidism and infectious process.

Tolerance of this way of life implies that the *capacity for sacrifice* is a psychobiological element of psychosexual maturity, of the "genital personality." Mature human sexuality, after all, consists biologically in surrendering individuality in the sexual act, in surrendering sex cells, and in surrendering control over the children when they are ready for independence. The intrinsic relationship between psychosexual maturity and acceptance of sacrifice may explain why, in the group of patients with good prognosis, percepts of destruction were more frequent than in the group with bad prognosis. Apparently, a high level of self-awareness was conducive to more rigorous striving for re-establishing adequate interpersonal relationships, whereas 20 percent of the group with bad prognosis failed to form any percepts, resigned to unconscious symbiosis with the bacilli.

Before the introduction of chemotherapy, many of the poor-prognosis group stabilized themselves on this level in the protective world of the sanitarium. In 1956, Ferruccio Antonelli and Maria Seccia published a monograph on their experiences with 400 such patients whom they had motivated to end their love affairs with the disease and to resume constructive participation in human society. The authors made it clear that the establishment of an affectionate relationship between patients and physician played a strategic role in the shifts from disease to health.

3. The tendency to form percepts of the gray area at the top of the inkblot has two aspects that correspond to the psycho-biological behavior of tuberculosis patients:

   a) The area established the *final union* of the converging disjointed pairs of symmetrical inkblots and symbolizes the final goal of symbiotic and sexual striving: the overcoming of the frustrations and limitations inherent in the complicated coexistence of the many organisms that constitute the living stream of life. The tuberculosis patients' dominant genital motivation accounts for their surrender to the persons they love, even in cases where their own survival is at stake. Surrender should not be understood as necessarily demanding sexual acts. Those are only its biologically most obvious form. Basic is the mutual attraction of individuals who are carriers of the same recessive genes, which need each other to become biologically manifest. This attraction, however, also is manifest in non-sexual forms of behavior. L. Szondi (1948) convincingly documented that genes also account for individual choices of friends and of occupational associations. Their power in tuberculosis-prone individuals accounts for the latters' deep involvement in similarly motivated individuals, regardless of serious flaws of personality that frustrate the relationships and precipitate them into the regressive symbiosis with the Koch bacillus.

   b) The attention of tuberculosis patients to the highest point of the inkblot is in keeping with the common symbolism that identifies the lower levels with the physical, the higher levels with the psychic, sphere of existence. The attention of these patients to the highest level and their disregard of its broken end (cf. p. 109 ff.) is another expression of the observations made in connection with their percepts of Plate IV, #4 (p. 57) and Plate VI, #3 (p. 61): they reach psychically, imaginatively, beyond the physical limits of their existence.

As pointed out in the introductory analysis of this last plate of the series, its structure symbolizes *the end* of life in the double sense of the word: the *purpose* toward which the individual structure is directed, and the *death* which is the lot of all multicellular organisms. This basic scheme is perceived by every subject in forms that are in some respects isomorphic with their specific forms of healthy behavior and with the forms of their terminal disease.

Cancer patients perceive the inkblot picture, as well as their human environment, as a challenge to their capacity to control the objects of their dominant, most different, psychobiological function. Because their behavior has been guided since infancy by the instincts of self-preservation, their attitude toward the forms of the inkblots and of their environment has been characterized by a striving for control of their most highly valued objects. This endeavor has necessarily entailed diminished perceptiveness of the individual forms of the inkblots and of other personalities. They have unilaterally dealt only with those aspects of their environment that fitted their own vision, and have ignored the conflicting aspects of their objects. For instance, when Pope John XXIII conceived the revolutionary plan of the Second Vatican Council, he initiated it without prior consultation with either the Curia or anybody else, as he noted in his autobiography (1965).

When a cancer-prone individual experiences the irretrievable loss of the object that has been essential for his self-fulfillment, he becomes in Donne's phrase, his "own executioner", the organ that had expressed his dominant psychobiological need turning into the executioner's axe (Booth, 1975). Part of that organ's cells regress to the earliest level of life on which self-preservation and self-propagation are independent of oxygen, and thus they create the tumor, the object that cannot be lost but grows autonomously until it has destroyed all the less valued functions of living. Actually, the cancer cells are capable of surviving their body of origin ad infinitum if they are given adequate nutrition in a new host or a laboratory container. This ultimate resort of cancer patients is consistent with their disregard of the image of the end at the top of the last inkblot picture, and with their carelessness in matters of prophylaxis and therapy mentioned earlier in connection with Plate IV, #4 (p. 57). Unconsciously the cancer represents the object of their original striving and inspires resistance against its sacrifice. The decision to surrender the tumor to the medical profession confronts the patient with the existential question of whether he expects adequate satisfaction from the prolongation of a life that has lost its original objective. The lack of medical attention to this aspect of cancer therapy (Booth, 1973; Weinstock, 1974) explains why even the earliest and most radical operations often fail to cure the patients.

Tuberculosis patients perceive the inkblot picture and their human environment in the spirit of the "basic trust" they developed as infants, which allowed them to attain psychosexual maturity. Having started life as partners in the invisible dyadic bond with their mothers, they are aware of the many separations that characterize equally the last inkblot picture and individual existence in the world. The experience of the implied frustrations, however, does not disturb them, any more than secure infants or adults depend on constant physical reassurance that their mothers or mates continue to be theirs even when they are physically separated. In cases where tuberculosis-prone individuals do lose their mothers or their mates, their affectionate nature and symbiotic motivation often enable them to establish satisfactory substitute relationships.

Disease comes about when they have lost their mothers or their mates without the possibility of finding an adequate replacement. In these cases, the overwhelming symbiotic need finds compensation in surrender to life with the tuberculosis bacillus that eventually may end their physical existence. Nevertheless, the dyadic spirit of their infancy stays alive to the last and allows them to participate in existence cheerfully as long as the body permits. Keats expressed the final experience of the tuberculosis patient perfectly in his sonnet "Bright star, would I were steadfast as thou art," written in the terminal stage of his illness.

B. *Differentiation of Cervix Cancer and Lung Cancer in Plates IX and X*

In the course of the interpretation of the responses to Plate IX, I mentioned that in the group of genital cancers the incidence of tuberculosis criteria relative to lung cancer criteria was higher than the CA : TB ratio of 1 : 0.5 established for the two experimental groups. It was 1 : 0.87 in Plate IX and 1 : 0.6 in Plate X. These figures are particularly significant because the *over-all ratio of the cervix cancer group* was 1 : 0.3, proving that Plates I-VIII elicited very decisive cancer scores.

In order to clarify the difference in reactions of the lung cancer group and the cervix cancer group, a detailed comparison of their Rorschach records was undertaken. The following differences between the two groups were found:

(Cervix N=38, Lungs N=33; number of patients in percents.)

	Card	Cervix CA	Lung CA
1. Percepts of anatomical structures other than genital or respiratory organs	IX	15%	none
	X	28%	8% (3)
2. Percepts of genitals in cervix group, of respiratory organs in lung group	IX	23%	none
	X	26%	8% (3)
3. Percepts of containment of living organisms, water, or fire; e.g., seed pod, potted plant, aquarium, dammed-up water, fire in fireplace	IX	42%	none
	X	20%	none

Altogether, 85 percent of the cervix cancer patients gave one or more of the responses that differentiated them from the lung cancer patients. The following observations concerning these three types of responses may explain their psychological meaning:

1. General experience with the meaning of anatomical responses in the Rorschach test suggest that, in contrast to lung cancer patients, the cervix cancer patients are preoccupied with their own bodies, particularly with their genitals. This is understandable because, as mentioned earlier, these patients tend to be sexually frustrated.

2. Lung cancer patients in their Rorschach percepts very rarely manifest anxiety concerning their bodies, and very rarely concerning their lungs, although all but one of these particular patients had been aware of the localization of the disease and all but the first 15, of the nature of their illness. It is understandable that their percepts in respect of body consciousness differ so much from those of cervix patients. In contrast to the sexual needs of cervix cancer patients, the respiratory needs of the lungs are unconsciously satisfied as long as life lasts, and those who, like 90 percent of lung cancer patients, desire additional conscious satisfaction can easily obtain it from smoking cigarettes.

3. The third category of responses expresses strikingly the specific predicament of the cervix cancer patients. Their high motivation for sexual self-expression is kept confined to the pursuit of sex in the narrow contemporary sense of the word. The pregenital fixation of the personality generally prevents full integration of the sexual function in the self and in mature psychosexual

relationships. The conflicting motivations of ego and sex lead to the building up of tension, from which these patients seek release in depersonalized and frequently unsatisfactory genital activities (Chapter VIII, A). It may be mentioned that the percepts of the third sort sometimes symbolize a sequence of tension and release; e.g., a seed pod bursting open, a waterfall (four patients, in this study). Piotrowski (1957) interprets the percept of "water rushing through a canyon" as expressing a combination of sexual desire and resignation.

The fact that the sexual problem of cervix cancer patients manifests itself specifically in their reactions to the Rorschach Plates IX and X should be evaluated in the light of their responses to Plate VI, the "sex card." Here they react in the same manner as the other cancer patients (p. 93 ff): they rarely perceive the inkblot in terms of two interrelated objects, the way the tubercular do:

Clinical Diagnosis	Number	CA Type	No Trend	TB Type
Cervix Cancer	38	82%	15%	3%
Other Cancers	55	74.5%	20%	5.5%

The preceding figures suggest that, even when faced with the inkblot charged with sexual symbolism, cervix cancer patients form percepts that are determined by their pregenital personality organization rather than by their strong motivation for genital activity. The latter, obviously, is due to a constitutionally determined organ disposition that seeks autonomous satisfaction. In the absence of mature psychosexuality, the genital organs cannot serve their purpose of orgastic communication, any more than the loquacity of monomaniacal people can help their human relationships.

The response of cervix cancer patients to Plate VI confirms the idea that mere exposure to physical sexuality does not help the development of mature physical relationships between the sexes. Psychosexual maturity is the result of the affectional relationship of infant and mother prior to the differentiation of genital functions. The Masters and Johnson treatment of human sexual inadequacy (1970) owes its successes to awareness of the extragenital conditions of sexual love.

In contrast to Plate VI, the inkblot pictures IX and X are not weighted in the direction of sexual symbolism. It may therefore appear surprising that the last two Rorschach cards so frequently elicit from cervix cancer patients responses that reveal their sexual problem. The explanation of this seeming paradox is found in the demand character of the two cards. *Both* are weighted by their *coloring* in the direction of emotional stimulation and, therefore, are apt to mobilize the deep biological associations between emotions and sexuality.

Furthermore, Plates IX and X are most anxiety provoking for these patients. Plate IX has been found by several investigators of more than a thousand diagnostically mixed patients to be the most difficult one (Piotrowski, 1957), and Plate X is specifically difficult for cancer patients. As Kinsey found in his extensive sampling of the American population (1948, 1953), anxiety as such frequently causes sexual arousal, and cervix cancer patients are specifically liable to such a reaction, as mentioned above.

Plate X tests the subject by presenting symbolically the task of choosing his path into the future. It is evident from the clinical reports on cervix cancer patients that members of this group are likely to look into the future with apprehension that is due specifically to their problematical sexuality.

The comparison of cervix cancer and lung cancer in terms of Rorschach responses shows that this method helps on two levels in understanding cancer dynamics:

1. A *general predisposition* toward cancer is indicated in the prevalence of cancer criteria over tuberculosis criteria for the total score of all 10 cards.

2. Different *localizations* of cancer are reflected in specific types of responses; e.g., those which distinguished lung cancer and cervix cancer from each other. (There are too few Rorschach records from other clinical groups to be useful in differentiating their perceptanalytical and psychobiological characteristics. Individual records strongly suggest that research based on additional clinical material is promising.)

C. *Summary*

The preceding interpretations of the disease-specific percepts of the 10 Rorschach plates have been partly repetitious. The use of all 10 plates is analogous to the principle of taking x-ray pictures from several angles: often, only some of the exposures permit definite diagnostic conclusions.

There is another analogy between Rorschach exposures and x-ray pictures in the comparative study of cancer and tuberculosis: Given the common genetic disposition of the two diseases, the pathological process is determined by the relative penetrance of two alternative types of response under exposure to 10 existential situations. The Rorschach experiment showed that the disease character corresponds to the quantitative predominance of the disease-specific percepts. X-ray pictures of cancer patients often demonstrate that, at an earlier age, they had undergone a (usually subclinical) tuberculosis infection. Various immunological and experimental observations make it likely that cancer should be classified as a metatuberculosis (Chapter V, A). As mentioned earlier (Chapter II, C), about 10 percent of tuberculosis patients end as cancer patients. The dynamics of this change will be discussed in Chapter V.

The following summary juxtaposes seven characteristic forms in which the respective disease predispositions of cancer and of tuberculosis patients manifest themselves in their percepts of the Rorschach plates and in their actual behavior. (The figures in brackets following each definition refer to the plate and to the criteria from which the particular common denominator was abstracted.)

CANCER	TUBERCULOSIS
Self-expression	
is favored by isolation from equals (IV, 1-3; V; VIII,2) and discouraged by their presence (VII,1; IX,2,3)	is favored by the presence of equals (I,1; II,2; III,1; VII,1; IX,2,3) and discouraged by their absence (IV, 1-4; V; VII,2; X)
The attitude toward the environment	
is *consistent* because the strong individualistic bias permits only one choice among multiple possibilities inherent in the same situation (II,3; III,4; VIII,3)	is *inconsistent* on account of openness to the multiple possibilities inherent in the same reality situation (II,3; III,4; VIII,3)
External difficulties	
are *ignored* regardless of consequences for achievement in order to maintain a consistent individualistic course throughout life (I,1-2; II,1,2; III,2; IV,1-4; V; VII,1,2; VIII,2; X,1,2)	*influence* the course of life as they lead to avoidance reactions and search for favorable conditions (II,1; IV,1-4; VII,2; VIII,2; X,1,2)

Interpersonal relationships

a) *socially* are experienced as *coexistence of autonomous* individuals (II,2; III,1,2; VII,2)

b) *sexually,* the *autonomy* of male and female is emphasized, the mate is experienced as an object, not a partner (VI,2)

a) *socially* are experienced as *interdependency* (I,1; II,2; III,1,2; VII,1)

b) *sexually,* the differences between male and female are subordinated to the experience of the mutual *interdependence* of mates (VI,2)

Appeal to emotions and sensuality

tends to be ignored or minimized. Self-destructive reactions are apt to result (III,3; VI,1; VIII,1; IX,1-3)

finds an easy response and stimulates a constructive attitude (III,3; VI,1; VIII,1; IX,1-3)

Self-revelation

is avoided as defense against involvement with others. Inner attitudes are hidden behind a noncommital social role (I,3; VII,1,2)

is used exhibitionistically in order to establish interpersonal relationships even if it involves the disclosure of weakness (I,3; VII,1,2; X,2)

Anxiety

results whenever the need for *autonomy is threatened* by social situations that demand interaction with equals (II,2; III,1; VII,1; IX,2,3). The subject *withdraws,* even fights (II,2; III,1), and reality perception becomes dedifferentiated and concretized (VII,1,2; X,1,2)

results when an existing, satisfactory *symbiotic relationship is lost* without an adequate substitute in sight (IV; V; VII,2; X,2). Feeling desperate, the subject *reaches out* for inadequate symbionts, imagination filling the gap between need and reality (IV,4; VI,3; X,3)

IV

The Isomorphism of Rorschach Percepts and Somatic Dynamics

The preceding chapter ended with the description of the two situations that cancer and tuberculosis patients, respectively, experience as a threat to their existence. Even if the threat is merely symbolized by the gestalt of the particular inkblot, enough anxiety is created to provoke specific percepts, which reveal specific risks of regressive behavior even in the absence of physical disease. Whereas such behavior is reversible in healthy subjects, it takes the form of somatic regression when the reality situation overtaxes the frustration tolerance of the organism. Incapable of actualizing its gestalt tendency on the level of interpersonal relationships, the organism is reduced to self-expression on a more primitive, cellular level.

The following juxtaposition of the pathophysiology on cancer and on tuberculosis, respectively, shows that the behavior of the diseased tissues is isomorphic with the gestalt tendencies manifest in the Rorschach percepts.

CANCER	TUBERCULOSIS
The organ mediating the dominant organ function of the subject (Chapters V, VI, IX) compensates for the *loss of control* over its external object by trans-	The organism compensates for the *loss of a symbiotic partner* by substituting the more primitive, and formerly ubiquitous, mycobacterium tuberculosis. Since

forming part of its own cells into the tumor, an internal object that cannot be lost (Booth, 1965, 1969b). This symbolic preservation of the lost external object is enhanced on the cellular level by regression of the metabolism from dependency on oxygen respiration to the phylogenetically more primitive process of fermentation. The latter sacrifices differentiation, but gains superior survival capacity for the unconscious substitute of the lost original object (Warburg, 1956, 1964). In other words, a person dies from cancer after having exhausted his vitality up to the very end in the creation of the tumor, unless causal therapy intervenes (Chapter IX).

these patients experience physical survival without a congenial partner as valueless, the organism surrenders to the bacterium. This surrender, however, is conditional. Thanks to their "eternal hopefulness," the tuberculous maintain to the last the capacity to switch their symbiotic needs back from the bacillus to human partners until their vitality is completely exhausted. A person dies from tuberculosis when the body has been consumed in the fatal symbiosis with the bacillus. The most vital concern of life has been relatedness *between* the own and other organisms; in isolation the own body has no value.

The novelist, Charles Dickens, expressed the body-transcending character of tuberculosis so well, that back in 1920 Friedrich von Mueller, an extremely "scientific" internist, quoted in his standard textbook these lines from "Nicholas Nickelby:

> There is a dread disease in which the struggle between soul and body is so gradual, quiet and solemn, and the result so sure, that day by day, and grain by grain, the mortal part wastes and withers away, so that the spirit grows light and sanguine with its lightening load.

In cancer, the opposite happens. The diseased organ grows and becomes heavier, and the patient becomes more depressed as he/she perseveres to the very end of his life in the struggle to express concretely his/her dominant organ function. It is this *concreteness and inflexibility* that so easily lead to an experience of "irretrievable loss." They result in the "brittle object relationships" that Elida Evans noted (1926) in the first modern monograph on the psychology of 10 cancer patients.

The lives of Napoleon I and Pope John XXIII, both victims of stomach cancer, illustrate how "neoplastic personalities" pursue their highly specific, individual goals in a self-absorbed manner, paying little attention to disturbing and even destructive consequences for themselves or for others.

Napoleon I considered his famous military campaigns as merely incidental to the fulfillment of his plans for the political and legal unification of Europe. Thus, he did not seek a soldier's death at Waterloo, but honorable asylum in England, his most persistent enemy. Cancer killed him, not after the loss of his political power, but after he had prepared for posterity an account of his constructive achievements and plans. Today, 150 years later, it has become evident that as administrator and legislator he did indeed make an enduring contribution to modern France and to the progressive unification of the western world.

Pope John XXIII in 1965 gave the ecumenical ideals of the Church a concrete form by calling the Vatican Council and inviting observers from other denominations. He made this decision without giving any thought to the foreseeable conflicts with the powerful conservative faction of his clergy. He died after he had found himself incapable of making the Council move according to his expectations.

These two highly intelligent, vital, and, in many respects, flexible personalities illustrate most strikingly the demonic *power of the rigidly conceived dominant object* of the neoplastic personality as it manifests itself consistently in the Rorschach percepts of the unselected patients who were the subjects of this study. This point is supported by the research of Miriam Shrifte (1962), who used the classical method of Rorschach analysis in a comparative study of the prognosis of cancer patients without knowledge of my then unpublished findings. Shrifte made the seemingly paradoxical discovery that the prognosis is *negatively related* to the creative endowment of the patient. She concluded that "if an individual's investment in moving is stronger than his capacity to be moved [this results in] processes of unproductive wasted vitality" which favor the growth of cancer.

This formulation agrees with my concept of the rigidity of the dominant object relationship. Since cancer patients cannot relinquish their investment in the external object after its loss, they are forced to waste their vitality, at the rate of its strength, in unconsciously producing the immovable internal substitute. Shrifte herself interpreted her findings in terms of "host resistance," a concept I consider inapplicable in view of the fact that the tumor develops from the cells of the organism itself.

The perceptanalytical study of cancer has made it clear that the disease can be understood only if it is considered as the result of the interaction between a specific personality type and the impact of a specific experience this type cannot cope with. Personality and experience can take many different forms, depending on the variations of individual biological and psychological endowment. The variations determine the sphere of existence in which the given subject is most vulnerable.

Since in so many respects cancer patients are very unlike each other, the concept of a "cancer personality" has met with great resistance from the majority of modern, somatically indoctrinated physicians. Their disbelief has been aided and abetted by the characteristic secretiveness of cancer patients in respect of their most vital concerns. Even psychiatrists are often deceived by the glaring, but superficial, dissimilarities between the patients, and by their overt behavior. Sometimes when I have delivered papers on cancer, colleagues have challenged me in the discussion afterwards, mentioning cancer victims they thought proved my concepts wrong. In many instances I realized they were ignorant of facts that I knew at first hand but did not have the right to reveal.

As far as the validity of my perceptanalytical criteria is concerned, no criticism based on their application has been forthcoming, although I have made them available since 1964 to some skeptical psychologists who have access to cancer patients. Since 1974, thanks to the initiative of Charles Weinstock (1974), I have had the opportunity of examining a growing number of Rorschach records taken by interested colleagues. None of them has yet given me cause to revise my criteria.

The psychological interpretation of the Rorschach criteria was developed from records administered by others and analyzed by me prior to any extended personal contacts with cancer and tuberculosis patients. This proved to be an approach I strongly recommend to those who plan to apply the Rorschach method to other clinical research. The independently recorded perceptanalytical data exploded various preconceived hunches that might have misled me if I had started working with patients of my own. Having learned beforehand from these records the nature of the psychodynamically significant situations, I was enabled to direct my inquiries toward those areas and to use the patients' personal imagery as a means of eliciting specific information. As I pointed out in earlier publications (Booth, 1958b, 1963a, 1963b), reticent subjects generally find it much easier to reveal themselves by explaining their own imagery than by answering abstract questions concerning their feelings and experiences.[8]

Confirmation of my interpretation of the psychodynamics of cancer and tuberculosis came, not only from my patients, but also from cancer patients I had personally known well as friends and relatives, and from published biographical and autobiographical accounts, among them: Sir Francis Chichester (1964), John Gunther Jr. (Gunther Sr., 1949), Brian Hession (1957), Pope John XXIII (1965), Gerard Philipe (A. Philipe, 1963), and Ludwig Wittgenstein (Malcolm, 1958). An outstanding document of self-revelation and of patient observations is Alexander Solzhenitsyn's autobiographical *Cancer Ward* (1969). Most of these accounts were given by individuals who had no knowledge of any psychologic concepts of cancer; some others, by colleagues opposed to such concepts. In this respect, the biographies of Signund Freud by Ernest Jones (1953, 1957) and by Max Schur (1972) are particularly illuminating (Booth, 1973).

In concluding this rather lengthy exposition of Rorschach findings in cancer and tuberculosis, the most significant results may be pointed out:

1. The core problem of these patients is constitutional and manifests itself throughout life in a specific way of perceiving their human environment.

2. The nature of this bias is manifest in the gestalt tendencies of their inkblot percepts.

3. If the reality situation frustrates the dominant constitutional need of the subject to an intolerable extent, the need finds expression in the form of regressive cellular changes.

4. Therapy is rational only if it includes a clear understanding of the frustrating situation and attempts to change it. Even total destruction of all tumor cells is only an emergency measure, very much like first aid in cases of serious suicidal events. The patient remains cancer prone, and prophylaxis of recurrences must be based on finding an acceptable solution of his psycho-social impasse (see Chapter IX).

5. Particularly in the case of the constitutionally reticent cancer patient, the Rorschach method can be helpful in spotting the nature of the problem because the 10 inkblots are focused on 10 specific forms of potential conflict. The formal score and the contents of the percepts are apt to guide the psychological approach on the part of the physician who is aware of the psychodynamics of cancer (cf. Chapter IX).

6. The problems of cancer patients are an integral part of the social forces which shaped their infantile environment and their adult opportunities for self-fulfillment.

The second part of this investigation will elaborate the theoretical and practical implications of the new perspectives that have been opened by the insights provided by the Rorschach method. Their clinical significance may be anticipated in the light of the observations of René Dubos (1952) on the tuberculosis epidemic that preceded the present cancer epidemic. Dubos emphasized "the subtle interplay between the social body and the social disease" and saw the epidemic as "the consequence of gross defects of social organization, and of errors of individual behavior." He went on: "Man can eradicate it without vaccines and without drugs by integrating biological wisdom into social technology, into management of everyday life." Progress in this direction had required a shift of the public attitude "from the fear motive to the promotion of understanding."

Exactly the same statements are pertinent to the cancer problem, but *understanding* of the subtle interplay between the social body and the destructive behavior of cancer cells has been made particularly difficult in the course of the last 50 years. The period is characterized by total separation of its two most important medical developments: on the one hand, there has been the rise of psychosomatic medicine, recognizing the social factor in disease; on the other hand, Otto Warburg's discovery (1926) of the abnormal metabolism of cancer cells, for which he received the Nobel Prize, initiated an enormous concentration of research devoted to the study of cancer cells *in isolation from the organisms of origin.* The results of this unbiological approach necessarily intensified the fear motive, the myth of the "wild cell" that could develop in anybody and defy even the promptest and most thorough therapeutic measures.

At the present time, understanding of the cancer problem is made extraordinarily difficult by the alienation between the two indispensable branches of scientific medicine. They cannot communicate because biological medicine speaks the language of animate behavior whereas molecular medicine speaks the language of "the all-embracing physical laws of inanimate matter." The quotation is taken from Hans Selye's plea (1967) for the integration of the important findings of molecular biology into those of "supramolecular biology." Selye's perspective, which inspired his Nobel Prize-winning work on stress, is based on his love of *"life itself as manifested by form*—things I can appreciate directly with my senses."

Form is, after all, the medium of communication on which life has been depending from its very beginning, millions of years before mankind developed languages. Words have been serving specifically human needs of differentiated communication, but they all too often have proven fallible and misleading because man's pioneering spirit is inclined to formulate limited perceptions of the mysteries of nature prematurely, and to freeze them.

Cancer is one of the phenomena which have been obscured by premature verbalizations of partial scientific insights. The Rorschach method avoids these pitfalls and makes it possible for cancer patients to communicate the forms in which they experience their life situations. The analysis of their percepts reveals the gestalt of the organism-environment unit that is subject to the disease, and the conditions that lead to self-expression in the form of cancer.

Seen in this psychobiological perspective, cancer can be rationally understood as one of the vicissitudes of the human experiences of finitude. This knowledge eliminates the unreasoning fear of cancer as a mysterious demon likely to attack anybody out of the blue, and should put an end to the current squandering of minds and monies on the utopian idea of "eradicating cancer in our time." The psychobiological concept of the personalities of cancer patients does not make such extravagant claims, but the following chapters will show that the humanistic consideration of the life situation of the patient can improve the results of somatic therapies, and that understanding of the psychosocial background of the epidemic may reduce the risks for future generations.

PART II

ANTHROPOLOGICAL ASPECTS OF THE CANCER EPIDEMIC

V

The Psychobiological Development
of Cancer Patients

"Physiological isolation, with its many causes, may well
be the most important single factor predisposing to the
reassertion of that life force to which, in certain circumstances, we give the name of cancer."
                                                                  —*D.W. Smithers (1964)*

A.   *Genetic Vulnerability and Traumatic Infancy*

The epidemiological research of Cherry (1924, 1925) and of
Haybittle (1963) has provided conclusive evidence that *cancer is a
risk limited to the nearly 20 percent of Caucasian populations who before 1850 had predominantly become victims of tuberculosis and
rarely developed cancer.* Since 1850, a steady change of morbidity
has been taking place: the incidence of tuberculosis has declined at the
same rate at which the incidence of cancer has increased. At the
present time, tuberculosis has become as rare as cancer was before
1850.

For a long time this change remained unexplained. René and Jean
Dubos pointed out (1952) that the tuberculosis epidemic had begun to
recede more than 30 years before Robert Koch identified the bacterium
and the medical profession reluctantly accepted the infectious nature of
the disease. The explanation occurred to me in 1967, when I realized

that there were three well-known medical facts that fitted together like pieces of a very simple jigsaw puzzle, yet had never previously been brought together:

1. Since 1958 (Booth, 1964b, 1965), I had known from my Rorschach investigation that the personalities of tuberculosis and of cancer patients differed consistently in respect of their psychosexual character traits; tuberculosis patients are genital characters (Abraham, 1925), cancer patients are anal characters (Freud, 1909) (see Chapters II-IV).

2. Since 1945, I had followed the work of Spitz (1965) on infantile development and known that the fixation of the psychosexual development on the pregenital level (e.g., anal fixations) is the result of a disturbance of the dyadic infant-mother relationship in the first year of life.

3. Since 1960, I had known from the work of Joseph Berkson about Cherry's discovery that since 1850 cancer had begun to replace tuberculosis.

The conclusion was inevitable: since 1850, a steadily increasing number of individuals developed cancer, starting with those who had been infants around the turn of the century. This was the time in which the Industrial Revolution gained momentum and forced many proletarian mothers to return to the factory after giving birth, leaving their babies to be hand-fed by others. At first, most of the infants died, but gradually the procedure became more successful, particularly after 1845, when the rubber nipple was invented, and when medicine improved nursing formulas and hygiene. Around 1890, the survival rates of bottle babies and breast babies became even.

The growing popularity of bottle feeding and the spreading of cancer went on side-by-side without anybody's thinking of a connection. Everybody was convinced that modern pediatrics, and particularly bottle feeding, were a great success. Even when Spitz, one hundred years after the invention of the rubber nipple, emphasized the fact that infants have important needs for affectionate contact with the mother, the attitude of physicians and of the general public remained complacent. I myself, obviously, had for several years not drawn the painful conclusion that the cancer epidemic is, to a considerable extent, caused by callous treatment of *sensitive* babies. A certain amount of unaffectionate treatment of babies has obviously always existed. Since 1973, the "History of Childhood Quarterly—The Journal of Psychohistory" has systematically collected evidence in addition to the earlier research (Am. Hum. Assoc., 1963; Nat. Society, 1959-1966; Rusk, 1966; Schloesser,

1964). These cases, however, had been individual aberrations of instinct, whereas artificial feeding became institutionalized frustration of infants (cf. Booth, 1975).

Readers of the preceding chapter will remember that, genetically, tuberculosis-prone babies are born with an abnormally great need for affection. They, therefore, are at high risk to experience frustration if they are nursed in a depersonalized manner. This happens most easily in bottle feeding, but breast feeding is not a solution for those modern mothers who feel awkward about "serving as cows" (Booth, 1967b, 1969b). My conclusion, that the intensity of the infant's need for affectionate nursing has a decisive genetic determinant, had been based originally on theoretical reasoning. Recently, Samuel Abrams and Peter Neubauer (1975) have provided empirical confirmation based on longitudinal observations of infants. They found that the primary orientation of infants toward the environment is either *human oriented* or *thing oriented.* For a *thing-oriented* infant, obviously breast and bottle are readily interchangeable, since both appease hunger; whereas for the *human-oriented* infant, the affectionate interaction with the mother's body is radically different from sucking a rubber nipple.

The distinction between the two genetic groups obviously does not deny that *human-oriented* infants can be damaged by inadequate feeding, and that *object-oriented* infants can be damaged by inadequate human contact; but it is important to realize that human health is primarily dependent on satisfaction of the individual's *genetically dominant need.*

In *thing-oriented* individuals, what dominates are psychobiological needs, which serve the purpose of *self-preservation.* In Chapter I (pp. 11-13), I described the L-type and the V-type which represent, respectively, dominance of the locomotor and of the cardiovascular system. Both are clearly *thing-oriented:* they secure the food and shelter that are essential for individual survival and only secondarily involve interpersonal relationships. They are compatible with a Robinson Crusoe existence.

In *human-oriented* individuals, *psychosexual needs* are dominant. They serve the *preservation of the race* and depend on interpersonal relationships. The biological core of the sexual act is embedded in the differentiated evolution of affectionate bonding and of the family. The description of the tuberculosis-prone personality type pointed out that these individuals are apt to neglect their own survival needs in the pursuit of love and sexual passion as well as in the mothering function. Sex and mothering together constitute the biological sphere that underlies the *human-oriented* personality type. As the Newtons (1967) formulated it: "The survival of the human race, long before the concept of 'duty' evolved, depended upon the satisfaction of the two voluntary acts of reproduction—coitus and breast feeding. These had to be sufficiently pleasurable to ensure their frequent occurrence."

Since the individualism of the industrial age has imposed its frustrations upon many genetically *human-oriented* mothers, the consequence is that their babies have become *secondarily thing-oriented*. If they survived at all, the babies did so because their oral and anal survival functions received adequate support and vicariously satisfied their crippled need for dyadic intimacy with the mother. Since they could not develop emotional security based on genetically intended mutuality, anxiety created the need for control of their objects. Winnicott's "transitional objects" (1953) became permanent elements of their lives. Those who have read earlier studies of cancer personalities (Evans, 1926; LeShan and Worthington, 1956) will find in them many illustrations of the general conclusion, that the object relationships of later cancer patients are generally highly personalized. In other words, these persons pursue control of specific objects with the intensity of lovers, in contrast to primarily *thing-oriented* individuals. For the L- and V-types, the exercise of their dominant psychobiological survival function is vital, and they can change their objectives; the activist, between different occupations and sports; the conformist, between different employments and leisurely retirement.

Cancer-prone personalities are different. They feel themselves into their objects so that they become part of them (Evans, 1926). "The self appears to be seen in a basically 'all-or-none' manner. It can break, but not bend" (LeShan, 1966). The intensity of their commitment to their chosen way of life makes them usually healthy, down-to-earth individualists. To all outside appearances, they have successfully survived inadequate mothering and often additional traumatic childhood experiences, as LeShan and Worthington (1956) and many other observers noticed.

The expression "traumatic" should be qualified, since it depends on the personality whether certain blows of fate are damaging. If one considers that cancer-prone subjects survive the frustration of their congenital human-oriented needs, and generally are very healthy prior to cancer, one realizes that they have been endowed with *superior vitality*. Their pregenital fixations prevent them from spending their energies in the passionate interpersonal involvements that are the special risk of the human-oriented individual. Thus, they are forced to develop the virtues of the anal character. To be "parsimonious, orderly, and obstinate" (Freud, 1909) means that they are self-sufficient. Thus they can take in their stride misfortunes that would precipitate less vital subjects into somatic or psychological invalidism and death. Seen in this light, the early misfortunes of adult cancer patients testify to the strength they successfully invested in their individualistic way of life, the substitute of the dyadic life style of the genital character.

B. The Carcinogenic Trauma

There has been ample documentation of the fact that cancer develops after the experience of having irretrievably lost an object that had provided vital satisfaction for the cancer-prone subject, as explained above (LeShan and Worthington, 1956). In many cases, the loss is brought about by a death, a divorce, or a career failure, events that frequently become public knowledge. In some cases, however, the loss remains a secret, because cancer patients are notoriously shy of self-revelation (Abrams and Finesinger, 1953; Goldsen et al., 1957; Kissen, 1963; Booth, 1965). The following example from my own practice may illustrate this point:

Miss Hope, aged 35, had been working for 10 years as editor for a famous scientist-author when she entered psychotherapy on account of a deep depression. Fourteen months of a seemingly very frank and trusting exploration of her situation provided neither an explanation nor a cure. She quit her job and two weeks later she developed a temperature and slight cough. An operable lung cancer was promptly discovered, but for six weeks she delayed surgery. By then, the tumor had become inoperable.

On the anniversary of Miss Hope's death, her closest woman friend visited me "to make a confession." Miss Hope had for several years pursued the plan of seducing the author, who had flirted with her very freely but refused to have intercourse. Miss Hope finally enlisted her friend's help to turn her birthday party into a threesome orgy, playing on the author's well-known sadistic and voyeuristic inclination. He cheerfully participated, but did not perform intercourse. Miss Hope felt deeply humiliated, and nine days later the cancer became manifest.

Aside from obvious traumatic experiences, frequently the loss of the vital object develops in ways that are more difficult to identify because they come about gradually. The popular concept of "cancer age" is based on the observation that the physiological process of *aging* reduces the capacity of everybody to maintain control of one's objects and way of life. As pointed out, the object that is vital for the cancer-prone subject is specific. Because it takes the place of the frustrated striving for a sexual mate, it is highly personalized, the object of the genetically dominant psychobiological function. The dominant-object relationship is very different in tuberculosis, where the subject's infancy had permitted the psychosexual development to reach the genital level. As documented in the preceding chapter, tuberculosis patients generally are not possessive, but apt to replace a lost love object when they find a congenial human substitute. In case this is not possible, they become tuberculous, remaining within the basic genetic orientation. Man and bacillus are both animate, and clinical experience shows that tuberculosis patients readily abandon symbiosis with the bacillus when they find a human mate who satisfies their sexual and/or emotional need.

The repressed *genital element in the dominant object of cancer-prone subjects* is most evident in the fact that aging, with its declining sexual motivation, often turns tuberculosis into cancer: in 5 to 6 percent of skin localization (Schwartz, 1960) and in lung tuberculosis, an increasing number of such observations has been published in recent decades (Gerami and Cole, 1969). There is no anatomical evidence that tubercular lesions *cause* cancer (Schwartz, 1960; Greenburg et al., 1964). The *cancerogenic effect of aging* has also been evident in ulcerative colitis (Fullerton et al., 1962) and is common knowledge in peptic ulcer, both diseases that share with tuberculosis the personality trait of being very dependent on personal support. The conclusion suggests itself that *sex hormones* support the human orientation and that their declining role favors pregenital motivations. This is in keeping with the experience that older people often develop more pronounced anal character traits: parsimony turns into miserliness, punctuality into an obsession with time schedules, and obstinacy into inflexibility.

The cancer-inhibiting role of sex hormones seems also evident in the fact that leukemia is the leading disease causing death in childhood, particularly in boys five to nine years old. Only accidents take a higher toll. Since "cancer was not even listed among the 10 most frequent causes of death in children" until 1940 (Ariel and Pack, 1960), the usual explanation appears unconvincing; that is, that all the former mortal diseases of children have been brought under control, leaving cancer as their leading risk. Why did childhood leukemia not stay a rare disease? The most plausible explanation seems to be that the incidence of inadequate mothering has risen from generation to generation for reasons discussed in Chapter VII, B, C. Consequently, congenitally human-directed infants are more frequently being traumatized. This theoretical inference is empirically supported by the careful clinical observations of Green and Miller (1958), who also have surveyed supporting evidence from the literature: that the mothers of leukemia victims often are inadequate, often themselves had experienced inadequate mothering (Bozeman et al., 1955; Orbach et al., 1955). The high sensitivity of leukemia infants in respect to the quality of mothering they receive is particularly documented by the fact that, of pairs of homozygotic twins, usually only one develops leukemia. Mothers of such homozygotic twins generally favor one, and it is apparently the relatively rejected one who gets the disease. Children obviously do not enjoy the benefit of hormonal compensation that makes cancer most infrequent in the age span between 15 and 25 (U.S. Public Health Service, 1974), when biological sexuality is at its highest level.

In older patients, the highest cancer incidence clearly coincides with the ages in which the psychosocial situation makes it most frequently difficult to replace the object of the dominant psychobiological function. This point will be discussed in the chapter on localization (Chapter VIII).

Some cases of cancer in creative personalities appear to be related to the experience of having exhausted their particular capacity for maintaining the activity that meant most to them. The brief biography of the philosopher Ludwig Wittgenstein by Norman Malcolm (1958) provides an extraordinarily clear picture of this type of development.

Wittgenstein had been an extremely lonely man. Leading the life of an "old spinster," he protected himself against the risk of having his feelings hurt, because he was extremely sensitive with respect to experiences in which people failed "even to be human." His lectures, however, provided him with the experience of intense human communication. They were completely unprepared, and developed, like Platonic dialogues, in spontaneous communication with the students, yet throughout their course he maintained an awe-inspiring control. For him, unlike most philosophers, reading and writing played a definitely secondary role in his life, and much of his teaching survives him only in two volumes of material which he had dictated to his students, and which for 10 years circulated privately among British philosophers.

Wittgenstein was considered "one of the most famous and influential philosophers of [his] time" when he resigned from his chair at Cambridge University at the age of 58. He gave as reason that he had become dissatisfied with his influence on the students. Evidently, the contact with students had been his vital object relationship. Having lost that, he tried to continue his research in utter loneliness except for the taming of wild birds. Thus he satisfied his genetic human-directed object need by regression to at least animate objects. Finally he arrived at the conclusion that he had "lost his talent for philosophy." At this time, about two years after his resignation, he developed cancer of the prostate, which killed him 15 months later. The diagnosis did not trouble him, but the fact that hormone treatment would prolong a life that no longer served a useful purpose. Actually, during the last two months of his life he was "apparently in the best of spirits," according to the biography. "As late as two days before his death he wrote down thoughts that are equal to the best he produced."

Wittgenstein's total commitment to one vital concern is a particularly convincing example of the object relationship of cancer-prone personalities, because he had proven outstanding gifts in many fields and commanded many opportunities for their exercise. A parable used by Wittgenstein to describe a man in a philosophical quandary illustrates the rigidity of the cancer-prone personality: "He is like a man in a room who wants to get out but doesn't know how to. He tries the window but it is too high. He tries the chimney but it is too narrow. If he would only turn around, he would see that the door has been open all the time."

Whereas in the case of Wittgenstein the loss of object control was due to the limit set by the declining vitality of age, in the case of the composer George Gershwin the limit was determined by the historical setting of his life. After a spectacular career as composer of popular music from the ages of 15 to 35, he went to Hollywood with the intention of financing a future as composer of serious music. But his life in Hollywood was ended abruptly by a brain tumor (astrocytoma of the right temporal lobe) which had, unaccountably, developed in the course of two years without being diagnosed.

In a discussion of the case in the New York Academy of Medicine (April 23, 1975), the musicologist Joan Peyser introjected the only pertinent psychobiological observation. She felt that Gershwin may have met a *timely* death, because the period (1937) was not favorable to serious music and he would not have been able to continue his career of public success. As a cancer-prone personality he was not endowed with the transcendental faith of Beethoven, who, when told on his deathbed that his last completed quartet had not pleased the audiences, replied, "It will please them some day."

C. The Psychobiological Meaning of Neoplasia

Freud very convincingly distinguished (1917) the psychological consequences of a vital-object loss for the pregenital and for the genital character as the difference between depression and mourning. He found that *in a depression the patient turns part of his own person into the lost object*. This process of introjection leads to the strange phenomenon that the depressed person makes great demands on the affection and concern of his environment but simultaneously condemns himself severely. The hostility, however, is actually not directed against the patient himself but against the original love object that disappointed him, and that he has introjected into his own self-image. This change of attitude toward the object from love to hate suggested to Freud that the object choice had been effected on a narcissistic basis to begin with. Thus, when obstacles arise in the way of object cathexis, the regression to manifest narcissism is inevitable.

As pointed out in the beginning of this chapter, the narcissistic satisfaction of the pregenital character is centered on *the experience of mastering the object*. The value of the object as such is reduced to that of an implement. The expendable quality of the original object of the anal function re-emerges in the self-debasing contents of the ruminations of the depressed patient. He compensates for the experience of injury and loss by indulging his ego in attacks on that part of his self which he has identified with the object. At the same time, he now has an object that cannot be lost, for it is now an integral part of the narcissistic ego and controlled by the ego. The demand for help is actually a challenge through which the ego tries to assert its power over his human environment.

Freud's description of the dynamics of psychological depression applies exactly to the process of cancer formation after the loss of an important object relationship. Instead of transforming part of the *psychological* personality, the *cancer patient transforms part of his body into an autonomous object that cannot be lost spontaneously*. It can be removed only by violent physical methods, with the exception of the rare cases of so-called spontaneous regression (Chapter IX). In spite of the mortal danger and of the deeply unconscious process of tumor formation, the cancer patient, like the psychologically depressed, tends to resist therapy. This behavior is particularly striking in the case of chronic cancer worriers (Goldsen et al., 1957).

The discovery that cancer patients experience the tumor as an anal object was made originally by Abrams and Finesinger (1953).

They found that the patients described their disease as "dirty, unclean, repellent, malodorous," and considered heart disease as "clean." The phenomenon was confirmed by Beatrix Cobb (1962). None of the authors seems to have been aware of the anal character structure of the pre-morbid personalities, but all were impressed by the association between guilt feelings and malignancy. Smithers (1964), whose biological cancer studies never touch psychodynamics, nevertheless considers this popular concept of "uncleanness" a major obstacle to rational cancer therapy: "The removal of the public fear and *shame* [italics mine] ... is in itself of great importance and alone worth working for."

It is very illuminating to observe that Freud himself was extremely reluctant to consider the importance of the anal character structure in depression. Contrary to his habitual concreteness in referring to the infantile roots of adult human behavior, he describes the melancholiac in terms that are applicable to a child who has failed to master bowel movement, but says it indirectly (Freud, 1917). Instead of referring to the child's shame over not having been "good," he writes about the "dissatisfaction with the self on moral grounds [being] by far the most outstanding feature." Instead of referring to the soiled child's calling for help, he notes that "shame before others... is lacking in him, or at least there is little sign of it. One could almost say that the opposite trait of insistent talking about himself and pleasure in the consequent exposure of himself predominates in the melancholiac." Freud explains this behavior as "plaints" in the legal sense of the word: "It is because everything derogatory that [depressed patients] say of themselves at bottom [sic!] relates to someone else that they are not ashamed and do not hide their heads." If one substitutes for "someone else" the fecal mass at the infant's bottom, it is evident that the only recourse against the condition is the drawing of attention to one's self by means of the voice. "The self-accusations of the melancholiac are hardly at all applicable to the patient himself ... but are reproaches against a loved object which have been shifted onto the patient's own ego .... The shadow of the object fell on the ego." On the infantile level: the fecal mass is reproached for having escaped the control of the anus. It provokes the sadistic reaction with its threat of suicide in which "*the ego is overwhelmed by the object.*"

Only following this sentence does Freud refer, in one brief paragraph, to the anal component. "We may expect to find the derivation of that *one* striking feature of melancholia, the manifestation of dread of poverty, in anal eroticism, torn out of its context [sic!] and altered by regression." The reluctance to consider the anal content of depression at all is even more evident in the original German formulation: "Es liegt denn doch nahe fuer den einen auffaelligen Charakter der Melancholie, das Hervortreten der Verarmungsangst, die Ableitung der aus ihren Verbindungen gerissenen und regressiv verwandelten Analerotik *zuzulassen* [= to admit]."

Freud's reticence in respect of the infantile situation behind the depressive fantasies is noteworthy. It suggests that the taboo of excrement is more severe than the taboo of sex. No wonder the unconscious resistance against the understanding of cancer psychodynamics is even greater than in the case of mere psychological depression. In cancer, there is a concrete and uncontrolled object in a place of the body where it should not be. As Abrams and Finesinger (1953) described it very clearly: "The discovery of the tumor is followed by the patients' reluctance to continue talking about themselves and their illness as freely as they had done before the nature of their illness was established." In other words, they behave as if they had become conscious of violating the anal taboo and try to ignore it because they are afraid of the rejection associated with infantile experiences of this sort. The interpretation is confirmed by the observation that those cancer patients who are told freely about their condition "are able to talk about their illness with ease and apparent satisfaction. They did not appear to suffer from the feelings of rejection noted in patients who had not been told or were unable to discuss their illness." Obviously, the physician who is capable of objectivity regarding cancer is one who does not react with irrational rejection to this disease.

Evidently, many people react on an unconscious level to the symbolical meaning of cancer which associates the uncontrolled growth with loss of bowel control. The latter, once a child has been toilet trained, becomes *an infantile expression of hostility* in case of disappointing parental behavior. The older child learns to substitute the word "shit" for the act, and most adults continue to use it, in thought or aloud, when they experience a failure to control a person or an object. Cancer patients, having lost the object of the dominant organ function, *curse somatically by creating the tumor in the frustrated organ*. Although in doing so they actually injure nobody but themselves, society reacts to this symbolical behavior as if they had defecated in public.

Some readers may think my emphasis on the anal taboo of cancer is excessive. A personal and general observation may serve as an explanation. In the early Sixties I offered a short book, containing the main observations and conclusions of the present volume, successively to 11 highly respected medical publishers. A number of them initially expressed great interest, but then withdrew their offers of a contract because their public relations advisers and sales managers had warned them against getting involved in this "controversial" subject. Several times the expression recurred, that they "would not touch it with a 10-foot pole." I finally realized that the unconscious association of money with excrement had made the financial advisers sensitive to the fact that the book would openly violate the taboo against undisguised anal display. Medical journals then provided decent privacy for publishing my "dirty" findings.

Recently Daniel S. Greenberg (1975), a highly respected science reporter, pointed out that after approximately two decades of the Federal "War on Cancer" and the expenditure of several billions of dollars, no significant progress has been made in dealing with the disease. He learned from some leading experts, who refused to let their names be known, that the money is spent on "dead-alley lines of research" and not on new ideas. When Greenberg inquired about one such project the National Cancer Institute had turned down, one of the top administrators advised him: "They're probably onto something pretty interesting, but it's really a bit too unconventional to expect this place to be interested in it." To put it briefly, billions of dollars are spent on research that promises to preserve the taboo of the human meaning of cancer. Molecular science is clean.

D. *The Biological Function of Neoplasia*

Understanding cancer as a somatized form of depression does not explain the self-destructive behavior of the introjected object. Although suicidal thoughts are common in depression, they rarely are carried out, and there seems to be general agreement that suicide among cancer patients is very rare in spite of their frequently tortured existence. That the organism should create out of its own cells the instrument of its death has given rise to the mythical language about cancer as an "invader," about the patient as "host," and about the "War Against Cancer." The paranoid attitude of the public is made graphic in Presidential proclamations and in the emblem of the American Cancer Society, which distorts the caduceus of healing into a blood-red sword.

In 1932 Henry Sigerist, the great historian of medicine, formulated the situation more soberly: "I personally have the feeling that the problem of cancer is not merely a biology and laboratory problem. But it belongs to a certain extent to the realm of philosophy. This, an X in the pathology of cancer, is a principle we do not understand yet. While we can understand most pathological processes as defense reactions or as healing processes, here we are facing a fact that does not fit at all into our general biological conceptions."

More than 40 years later these conceptions still prevail, which had developed under the influence of an individualistic and materialistic philosophy of life. They are, however, increasingly challenged by observations that human behavior is controlled only to a limited extent by conscious individual needs, and to a large extent by genetics and by unconscious psychological motivations. The cancer phenomenon illustrates this point.

In the beginning of this chapter I pointed out that the genetic orientation of these patients is characterized by the *dominance of the sexual instinct over the instinct of self-preservation*. This dominance has equally characterized the evolution of life as soon as organisms developed that were composed of specialized sex cells and body cells. For half a billion years, sex cells have secured the immortality of life by creating and abandoning mortal bodies.

In primitive plants and animals the organisms often die as soon as the birth of the next generation is secured. Evolution eventually obscured the basic principle when individual bodies became long-lived and animals differed in respect of their genetic orientation. Some individuals of a given species risk their lives in order to mate, others stay unmated but healthy if they cannot vanquish their rivals.

In the second section of the present chapter I described the infantile process that turns the innate sexual intensity of tuberculosis-prone subjects into the intense object relationship of the dominant psychobiological function. The irretrievable loss of the object thus represents a second, cumulative injury to the subject and results in the radical regression of neoplasia, the substitution of an internal for the external object.

The principle of this step was discovered 50 years ago and promptly rewarded with the Nobel Prize in 1930: Otto Warburg's demonstration (1926, 1956) that normal cells become cancer cells when they are deprived of the capacity to utilize oxygen and regress to the primordial process of energy production by fermentation. This change of metabolism is caused by chemical or physical agents which damage the *mitochondria*. These micro organs in the cell plasma became part of the animal cell after plant life had raised the oxygen content of the atmosphere far above the 1 percent level in the early stages of evolution. The utilization of oxygen by mitochondria has been an integral part of the morphological evolution of life and of the maintenance of cell differentiation. When deprivation of oxygen causes regression to energy production by fermentation, the cells continue to multiply, but on a morphologically inferior level.

Throughout his long life, Warburg (1967) insisted that "no disease exists whose primary cause is better known," viz., that all cancerogenic agents have in common the fact that they damage the respiratory function of the mitochondria; but unfortunately, because of his microbiological approach, he thought only in terms of chemistry and radiation. The observations of the psychobiological context of cancerogenesis suggests that a *functional disturbance of oxidation* may also be involved.

In the first place, the supply of oxygen to the body organs is regulated by the level of their activity. Thus it would be in keeping with physiological experience that the irretrievable loss of its object would reduce the blood supply to the dominant organ. In this respect, Warburg's observation of 1964 is significant: In embryonic chicken-cell cultures, cancer metabolism is induced by *low oxygen pressure*, but in the course of two cell divisions normal metabolism can be re-established by raising the oxygen pressure.

There is, furthermore, evidence that *shock* can injure the mitochondria and induce anaerobic metabolism (Schumer and Sperling, 1968). The latter factor may well play a major role in cases like the one mentioned above (Chapter V, B) and those where patients suddenly deteriorate after being told bluntly that they have cancer (Meerloo, 1954) without being offered more psychological support than the cold comfort that, according to statistical experience, a certain percentage of cancer cases survives (cf. Chapter IX).

The preceding observations on the nature of cancer cells suggest an explanation for the fact that cancer develops as a substitute object in the organ of the dominant psychobiological function. The following points are relevant:

1. The organism maintains its health as long as its vital organs can maintain at least a minimum of functional interaction with their specific environmental objects: oxygen, food, water, sensory input, and motor output. If this minimum is lost, the cells of the organ regress to a more primitive level of functioning.

2. In cancer-prone individuals, the dominant organ system requires a high level of functional interaction. On the human level of evolution, the oxygen metabolism of the organ cells

is an integral part of the object relationship of the organ system. Object-loss consequently reduces the oxygen supply to its cells to a lower level, the more so if there are also carcinogens involved. The cells survive their relative oxygen deprivation by regressing to fermentation as a source of energy. Thus they reactivate the primordial stage of evolution, when the forms of life were poorly differentiated but the single cells were endowed with the capacity for unlimited self-reproduction.

3. The metabolic regression of part of the genetically dominant organ system represents a biological over-compensation for the object-loss: inasmuch as cancer cells are endowed with virtual immortality.

4. The tumor is the internalized substitute for the lost external object. As pointed out in the beginning of this chapter, cancer-prone individuals are genetically programmed to be dominated by the need for an animate object; ideally, a sexual mate. The cancer is clearly a regressive form of an animate object and potentially immortal, like sex cells.

5. The analogy between sex cells and cancer cells is not limited to their potential immortality. Both also are unicellular organisms capable of leaving the tissue where they grew and of pursuing their specific biological programs: sex cells leave the gonads to secure the immortality of the species; cancer cells leave the organ of origin to create new tumors that perpetuate the survival of their morphological characteristics in other organs, or even, in case of transplantation, in the bodies of other members of the species. Sex cells and cancer cells are autonomous with respect to the organism in which they grow.

6. Cancer cells express the distortion of normal psychosexual development that takes place in infants who are genetically dominated by the sexual instinct but cannot reach the genital stage because of an inadequate nursing experience. The genetically dominant organ function, whether sex-related or not, becomes carrier of the crippled genital function. The cells of its organ, in becoming cancerous, assume the behavior of sex cells. The process is analogous to the *imprinting* of young animals. Hatching birds follow a person who was the first moving object they saw and become bonded to him rather than to the mother. The human infant, being biologi-

cally immature, apparently becomes easily imprinted by the experience of a mother who deviates from the physiological, dyadic behavior of the mother for which the infant is genetically programmed. The result is pregenital fixation of the sexual instinct, the dominance of oral and anal behavior in the eroticism of the adult.

Considering the fact that cancer patients are genetically dominated by the sexual instinct, the hypothesis deserves serious consideration, that inadequate mothering also imprints the disposition toward potential sexlike behavior on the cells of the dominant organ. This hypothesis is supported by the discovery that during the first months of life the testosterone level can reach half the values observed in adult men (Forest et al., 1973), and that in young female infants an analogous profile of estrogen levels has been observed. The authors of these studies drew the conclusion that the early temporary surge of sex hormones plays a role in the future life pattern of the adult. Apparently the close link between copulation and nursing emphasized by the Newtons (1967) has a hormonal component.

Summing up the preceding observations on the origin and nature of cancer cells: their destructive behavior against the healthy organism follows naturally from the fact that *cancer-prone individuals are genetically programmed for dominance of sexual motivation over the individual survival instinct.* Because their psychosexual development became distorted in the beginning of life, the relationship between their dominant organ function and its object became sexualized. Consequently, the loss of the beloved object caused part of the organ cells to regress to the primordial, presexual form of species survival, while sacrificing the body of origin.

On a regressive level, cancer patients enact the same life pattern as their genetic relatives, the tuberculosis-prone individuals. Having enjoyed the benefit of adequate mothering, the latter become dominated by the need for a satisfactory psychosexual relationship at the expense of their survival needs, and in case of frustration they regress to the partnership with the primitive bacterium tuberculosis. The bacteria, too, like cancer cells, have the capacity for unlimited reproduction.

Seen from the perspective of phylogenesis, neoplasia fits our general biological conceptions of pathological processes. Deprived of its normal object, the organism replaces it by way of regression to a phylogenetically more primitive level where at least two main elements of the genetic program find expression: cancer cells, like sex cells, potentially survive the rest of the organism, and they preserve morphological qualities of the cells of the organ in which they originated. Surveying the development of cancer patients through the vicissitudes of inadequate mothering displacement of sexuality to a specific organ-function, and the creation of the cancer, one must admire the tenacious self-assertion of specificity on the macro- and micro-biological levels of the individual. As Smithers (1964) clearly saw, the disease reasserts the life force that has been frustrated again and again by physiological isolation.

Once the deep psychobiological motivations of cancer patients, and their extraordinary vitality, are understood, it may be expected that fewer of the predisposed individuals will be forced to die of the disease in the isolation imposed on them by the current mindless concentration on destroying cancer cells without considering the human needs that created them. This point will be discussed in the chapter on therapy (Chapter IX).

E. The Life History of Sigmund Freud as a Cancer Patient

The preceding analysis of the psychobiological dynamics of cancer patients had to be rather general and could not do justice to the human drama that one finds in their biographies — if one succeeds in obtaining them. Instead of illustrating various points with anecdotal material, I shall confine myself to the life history of Sigmund Freud, which is unusually well known, thanks to the efforts of his biographers (Jones, 1953/57; Schur, 1972) and to his own psychological work which in many ways reflects his personality. The following points appear to be significant:

Freud was his mother's first-born child, after she had failed to conceive in the first five years of her marriage. She seems to have loved him particularly because a gypsy had predicted his brilliant future. There is reason to think that her affection involved a strong, possessive self-centered element. Throughout her long life she referred to her great son in the diminutive form of "her golden Sigi." Apparently she was very vain. Even in her 90's she resented the gift of a shawl and a photograph, because they made her look old. When she died at the age of 95, Freud experienced no grief because all his life he had been "terrified" by the fear that she might be hurt in case he should predecease her.

Freud was originally breast fed, but one does not know how long. It is certain that his mother became pregnant between two and five months after his birth (the two biographers contradict each other), and, given his mother's narcissism, one has reason to wonder whether she was adequately affectionate. Certainly Freud's exclusive intimacy with his mother was ended by the birth of his brother. Freud's self-analysis frequently mentioned his keen resentment of the intruder, although the infant died before Freud's second birthday, and he never overcame the trauma of his mother's "betrayal." Apparently his relationships with women were very inhibited. He married at the age of 30, after an engagement period of more than four years, and he lost all sexual responsiveness to women at 44.

At the same time, his pregenital fixation on orality was extraordinarily intense, suggesting that weaning had been premature. For enjoyment of living and for creative work, he depended on cigar smoking to such an extent that he could not abstain for long even during the last 16 years of his life, when smoking appeared to be an aggravating factor in his struggle with cancer of the right jaw.

The cancer developed when Freud was 67 years old. Apparently he had watched its growth for two months before he showed it to a colleague. The delay is as typical as the fact that at that time he faced the irretrievable loss of his most beloved grandchild, Heinele, who had contracted tuberculosis in the preceding year. The child had become "a bag of skin and bones." As a last desperate measure he underwent a tonsillectomy on April 20, 1923. This was the same day that Freud underwent his first cancer operation. Although his physicians had tried to deceive him about the diagnosis, Freud himself had no illusions. Nevertheless, he chose a mediocre surgeon, who performed in an outpatient department, and he did not even tell his family. His major concern seems to have been that he was warned against smoking.

Two months later Heinele died. "It was the only occasion when Freud was known to have shed tears. He told Marie Bonaparte that the blow was quite unbearable, much more than his own cancer." Three years later, when offering condolence to Ludwig Binswanger, whose eldest son had died, he said that Heinele had represented for him all his children and grandchildren, that since the child's death he had not been able to enjoy life. "It is the secret of my indifference—people call it courage—toward the danger to my own life." This is the account of Ernest Jones (1957).

Something more should be added to account for the deep involvement of the 67-year-old man with a 5-year-old child, even though he was "the most intelligent child [he] had ever encountered." In the light of the specific relationship between cancer and tuberculosis, the encounter between the cancer victim and the tuberculosis victim mobilized deeply unconscious problems.

In the course of Freud's life, the genital element in his personality had become increasingly repressed and depersonalized. Approaching sex from the point-of-view of his pregenitally fixated character, he had created in psychoanalysis a method of strengthening the control of the ego over the sexual instinct and over the object world. Seen in this individualistic perspective, sex had become—and to the end of his life, stayed—"a riddle" (1937). Anal self-sufficiency was incompatible with the dependency of biological sex on a partner. Erotic life involved a degradation of the ego (1908). Castration fear and penis envy appeared to Freud inescapable complications of sexual strivings, at least on the unconscious level. It is not surprising that as early as the age of 44 (Letter to Wilhelm Fliess of March 11, 1900) Freud's physical responsiveness to women had become completely repressed, but that on the psychological level his sexuality found continued expression in the psychoanalytical technique of letting his own unconscious tune in to the unconscious productions of his patients, and also in his intellectual concentration on the problem of sex. The impersonality of psychoanalytical practice and research safeguarded the ego against the threat of genital overvaluation of "the object."

In the case of Heinele, the defenses of Freud's ego against becoming overwhelmed by another person broke down. The male child did not represent the biologically re-enforced threat of feminine sex appeal against which Freud had become immune in the course of the past 23 years. Powerful attraction, however, was exercised by the strongly genital character of Heinele, proven by the fact that he became a victim of tuberculosis at an early age three years after his mother's death. In this "most intelligent child [he] ever encountered," Freud met with the alter ego of his own childhood, the genital potential of his personality, which the vicissitudes of his infancy had prevented from developing into a part of his adult relationships. That the potential must have been strong and been perceived as a threat to his need for ego control is implied in his irrational jealousies during his engagement years, and in the fact that sex was the focal point of his intellectual endeavors. At the age of 74 (Freud, 1930), he expressed the opinion that without sexual inhibitions there would be an end of all cultural endeavors. "What motive would induce man to put his sexual energy to other uses if by any disposal of it he could obtain fully satisfying pleasure? He would never let go of this pleasure and would make no further progress." This fantastic exaggeration of the power of biological sexuality indicates the intensity of the conflict between anal and sexual needs in Freud's basic personality make-up. The death of Heinele, representing his original genital endowment, dramatized the tragic outcome of Freud's struggle for integration of genitality in his personal life and in his scientific system. It was a vital object loss indeed that coincided with the beginning of his cancer.

The localization of the tumor in the oral region conforms with the general experience (cf. Chapter VIII) that neoplasia develops in the organ that mediated the dominant psychobiological function of the patient. That it was specifically the jaw suggests that there had been a strong aggressive component in Freud's fixation on his infantile weaning experience, which was acted out in his cigar addiction. On the last day of his life Freud provided impressive evidence of his self-understanding in the choice of the book he re-read: Balzac's novel "La Peau de Chagrin" (the title plays on the double meaning of "chagrin" that is missing in the English translation, "The Fatal Skin"). Freud commented on the appropriateness of the story as dealing with shrinking and starvation, but neither Jones nor Schur noticed that Freud's description was correct only in a symbolical sense. Actually, the conclusion of the book expressed Freud's lifelong fantasy of taking revenge on his mother in the most direct form: at the end of Balzac's romantic fairy tale the protagonist finds himself left with the magic power of having one last wish fulfilled. He achieves it in breaking down the locked door of his mistress, throwing himself on her, and *dying biting her breast.* What clearer communication could Freud have left behind, that he understood the cancer in his mouth as the substitute of his mother's breast?

F.   The Problems Obscuring the Understanding of Cancer Patients

The preceding biographical observations on cancer patients would not have surprised experienced physicians of old. They were well aware that cancer develops after the loss of an important emotional relationship in persons characterized as depression prone (Kowal, 1953; LeShan, 1959, 1965). Since the middle of the last century, however, physicians have become increasingly oblivious of the personality factors in disease because medical science has become possessed by the ambition to equal the spectacular progress of physics and chemistry. This meant that all healthy and pathological processes in the body were avidly studied with respect to those aspects that could be reduced to their molecular elements. A limitless faith developed that all diseases of body and mind were going to be cured by scientific manipulation of the body. Obviously, in the concept of man as a physico-chemical machine, there was no place for the old concept that health is decisively influenced by the spirit in which individuals meet the good and bad fortunes of their lives.

The vast majority of the public enthusiastically embraced the new faith, not only because it was new and simple. More important, it disposed of the old notions that people brought diseases upon themselves as punishments for having violated the laws of God or society or nature. Few are indeed the personalities willing to take responsibility for their own fate, particularly in matters of life and death. "Liberty means responsibility. That is why most men dread it" (G. B. Shaw).

Reduction of the cancer problem to the search for microscopic physico-chemical processes had obvious appeal for modern man. Faith in the infallibility of scientific method provided a socially respectable defense against subconscious misgivings that cancer might carry a human message. The intense need for this defense is reflected in the billions of dollars that institutions have continued to spend without significant medical success (cf. Chapter V, C) and in intellectual awareness that the cancer problems could not be reduced to a question of carcinogens. Even the Surgeon General's report of 1964 on "Smoking and Health" contained the admission, "Often the coexistence of several factors is required for the occurrence of a disease, and that one of the factors may play a determinant role; that is, *without it, the other factors (such as genetic susceptibility) seldom lead to the occurrence of the disease*" (U.S. Pub. Health Serv., 1964) (italics mine). The avoidance of one of the "other factors," psychodynamics, incidentally, is very evident in this report. Among the 189 consultants listed, only nine were psychologists, and *not a single one* of the numerous researchers who, since the early Fifties, had published psychosomatic studies sponsored by Harvard and other prestigious universities.

The role of the personal life history in cancer was further obscured by lapses of official language into a style of primitive animism reminiscent of preliterate demonology and magic. Presidents declare war against cancer, the American Cancer Society carries on "crusades" under the sign of a blood-red sword as substitute for the caduceus of medicine and promises to eradicate the ancient disease "in our time," the Government supports its materialistic philosophy by considering the successful moon shots as proof that the disease can be conquered by a colossal concentration of money and manpower. The equation of the mechanics of inanimate matter with living human beings does not make more sense than the preliterate medicine man's expecting to cure or kill people by manipulating their feces.

Science-minded moderns tend to rationalize their avoidance of the *human factor* by pointing out that in many respects cancer victims are very unlike each other. To mention such striking contrasts: Napoleon, the military conqueror, and Pope John XXIII, the apostle of ecumenical reconciliation, both died of cancer of the stomach; Senator Robert A. Taft Sr., who could not sell himself to his own party, and Arthur Godfrey, who can sell anything to anyone, both developed lung cancer, although the outcome was different (Wolters, 1959); Roentgen, the precise, sober physicist, and Freud, the adventurous theoretician of the psyche; John Foster Dulles, the proponent of "massive retaliation," and Rainer Maria Rilke, the hyperaesthetic poet; Leo Szilard, the versatile enthusiast for theoretical problem-solving (Rabinowitch, 1964), and Sir Francis Chichester, the "single-handed" sailor (Chichester, 1964); Ludwig Wittgenstein, the philosopher of language, who gave away his huge inheritance (Malcolm, 1958); and Damon Runyon, the cynical writer who said that "money is not everything, but 99 percent of everything" (Hoyt, 1964). Many readers probably can add to this list examples from personal experience. Actually all these contrasts prove only that all cancer patients share the same type of vulnerability, which they usually keep to themselves and only manifest in the symbolic language of the neoplasia.

The popular misconception of cancer as everybody's freakish physical risk is the unfortunate result of the molecular bias of modern medical research. Great intellectual efforts and vast economic resources succeeded in clarifying the microbiological processes by which specific chemicals and radiation transform the normal physiological behavior of cells into neoplastic behavior, behavior that characterized them regardless of the organ from which they had been taken.

No similar efforts were undertaken to elucidate the *biological conditions under which human beings and animals produce neoplasias.* The belief in the demonic power of carcinogens had such irrational hold on academic medicine that it was not shaken even when Richard Doll (Pike and Doll, 1965), one of the original apostles of the cigarette theory of lung cancer, recalculated his 10-year-old statistics a year after (!) the Surgeon General's report of 1964. Doll had to admit that no correlation exists between the length of time and the quantity of cigarettes the patients had smoked, on the one hand, and the onset of the disease, on the other. (For other aspects of this work, see Chapter VIII.) This climate of public and academic opinion left the field of psychosomatic cancer research to a few independent-minded individuals.

R. D. Passey (1962), one of the earliest workers in the field of carcinogens, epitomized his review of the irrationalities of this one-sided approach with a quotation from John Maynard Keynes (1936): "The difficulty lies not in new ideas, but in escaping from the old ones." One way of escape used in this investigation was originally proposed by Freud for the discovery of hidden meanings of the words of his patients: In cancer research one has to study the past and present of the individual subject with "evenly poised attention." There is good reason to expect that such effort will lead to awareness of the existential themes which give the life history of each patient its unique gestalt. Certainly, some cancer patients stick to their notorious secretiveness to the bitter end; but often enough their innate need for affection makes them open up to a physician who takes a genuine human interest in them.

VI

The Historical Development of the Cancerogenic Culture

A. The Psychobiological Concept of Culture

Apparently a collective aberration of human motivation is responsible for the epidemic rise of neoplasia among that part of the population which is genetically dominated by human-directed motivation (see Chapter V) and thus is most important for the future of mankind. In making this point, I am trusting that many readers share the view expressed by Konrad Lorenz (1966): "Far from seeing in man the irrevocable and unsurpassed image of God, I assert—more modestly and, I hope, in greater awe of Creation and its infinite possibilities—that the long-sought missing link between animals and the really humane being is ourselves."

There is certainly the biological possibility that the thing-oriented part of the population may eventually outbreed the human-oriented part. In this case the evolution of the human species would stabilize itself like that of the social insects who have not changed their social techniques of survival in the last 300-million years. On the other hand, however, are the biological observations emphasized by René Dubos (1965) that artificial population explosions lead to highly self-destructive social and sexual behavior, which reduces the population to a viable level. The survivors are descendants of the dominant and fertile individuals of the original population, whereas the descendants of the subordinate individuals have died out.

The current cancer epidemic alone—but, even more, the other social symptoms of an overpopulation crisis—calls for an historical perspective on its origin. This approach recognizes that the biological and social behavior of individuals is determined to an important extent by the gestalt of the society of which they constitute a part. We cannot undertake a rational approach to the cancer problem if we deal only with the symptom and its precipitation by factors that are not pathogenic for the majority of the population.

The declining intimacy between mother and infant since the beginning of the Industrial Revolution is an occidental trend that has run counter to the common feature of all other surviving cultures of mankind. Although many of them conceded to parents the right to kill unwanted children, they protected the physiological intimacy that infants need in the beginning of life. Before going into the circumstances that permitted the present population explosion in spite of unnatural forms of child care, it is important to clarify the historical development of the radical change in mothering.

The concept of human societies underlying the present chapter is an extension of the conclusions that Jakob von Uexküll drew (1921) from his biological studies of the inner and outer world of animals: "There are as many worlds as there are subjects. These subjective worlds are formed by limited numbers of spatial elements, movement patterns, time elements and qualities of content." Insofar as the subjects belong to the same species, their worlds are similar, but, even on a primitive level, by no means identical. The genetic and constitutional dispositions of animals determine, not only their bodies, but equally the worlds they are aware of. One may describe human constitutional types in the words used by Von Uexküll for animal species: "Independent organisms with their own characters and extremely long durations of life." The innate plan that connects the organism of the subject with selective elements of the environment accounts for the fact that perceptions of the 10 Rorschach plates reflect the psychobiological structure of the percipient. As Chapter III described in detail, the human psychobiological structure includes many social elements. It is more complex and rich than that of animals, but the basic fact applies to all: subjects perceive only those elements of "objective reality" that are isomorphic with their inner worlds.

The deterministic formulation of Von Uexküll's subject-environment unit was developed by Viktor von Weizsaecker (1940) into a psychodynamic concept of the basic principle. He followed Einstein's example and introduced the subject into his experimental designs by analyzing the interdependence of perception and motion in subject-object relationships. The investigations demonstrated that the popular stimulus-response concept is an illusion that is due to the nature of human consciousness. At any given moment we can be *aware* only of *either* perceiving or acting. In reality, subject and object interact simultaneously. Von Weizsaecker called this form of relationship *"Gestaltkreis"* (gestalt circle) in distinction to the linear stimulus-response concept. Introducing the gestalt concept, he acknowledged that visual perception involves a creative cerebral act, in contrast to the mechanistic idea that the optical system functions like a movie camera.

The discovery of the principle of the gestaltkreis led to the formulation which may be either expected or surprising because *"[biological] events are not linked by causality, but by decisions."* The future turns out to be "expected," that is, conforming to causalistic expectations, as long as the subject decides to keep a specific object-relationship static; the future turns out to be surprising whenever the subject decides to dissolve a specific form of subject-object coherence in order to create a new form, a new gestaltkreis.

The theory of the gestaltkreis is a simple and adequate description of the evolution of life. For some 600-million years, organisms maintained some basic elements unchanged (for instance, the cell as irreducible unit), yet the finer structures of cells underwent the most surprising and complex changes as they served the evolutionary changes of life. To realize that there is one underlying life process uniting subject and environment is to dispose of the conceptual awkwardness of theories of evolution that treat life as a linear chain of physico-chemical processes altered from time to time by *accidents*—surely an odd *deus ex machina* on the stage of science—such as gene mutations or environmental changes.

Although the existential biology of Von Weizsaecker does not bring us any closer to an understanding of the mystery of creation itself, it at least reminds biologists and physicians that they themselves are living parts of the processes they study, that they are challenged to make decisions *respecting the objects* of their studies, who are subjects as well. "Respecting" is used advisedly to emphasize the difference from the so-called "objective scientist" who, in hot pursuit of the "laws of nature," all too often forgets that the living organism is not a test tube, but a subject whose feeling-reactions influence the physico-chemical reactions to the experimental design. To strengthen the scientific basis of this remark, I shall quote from the Epilogue of "What

Is Life" (1945) in which the physicist Erwin Schroedinger drew the correct, noncontradictory conclusion from the following two premises:

"1. My body functions as a pure mechanism according to the Laws of Nature.

"2. Yet I know, by incontrovertible direct experience, that I am directing its motions, of which I foresee the effects, that may be fateful and all-important, in which case I feel and take full responsibility for them.

"The only possible inference from these two facts is, I think, that I — I in the widest meaning of the word, that is to say, every conscious mind that has ever said or felt 'I'—am the person, if any, who controls the 'motion of the atoms' according to the Laws of Nature."

In the light of all the preceding psychobiological considerations, respect for the actual and potential victims of the cancer epidemic demands that the psychobiological and cultural dimensions of the disease be understood. To clarify this point, it is necessary to consider other forms of disease from the same point of view.

B. Two Psychobiological Types: Hunters and Planters

In 1946, I published my comparative Rorschach study of the loco-motor and of the vasomotor personality types, which clarified the role of personality in the somatic disease processes that are the specific disease liabilities of these types (Booth, 1946b). Thirteen years later I was forcefully reminded of the archaic dimension of these earlier findings. Reading Joseph Campbell's (1959) book on the religions of primitive hunter and planter societies, I recognized, and Campbell confirmed to me, that the shapes of the artifacts of prehistoric hunters had turned up in the Rorschach percepts of modern arthritics and Parkinson patients so frequently that they made it possible to differentiate their Rorschach records from those of patients suffering from high blood pressure. The Rorschach imagery of the latter, in turn, recalled the artifacts of prehistoric planters. (See Appendix.) I may add that my descriptions of the behavior patterns of the two clinical personality types agreed with the descriptions Campbell gave of hunter and planter societies.

The specific character of the percepts of these two types is obviously based on the close symbiosis of the hunters with the animals on whom they preyed, and of the planters with the plants they cultivated. It is equally obvious that the two very different ways of life selectively bred two different psychobiological types fit for each one's survival. It is remarkable, however, that ten thousand and more years later the two genetic types have preserved, not only their specific value systems, but also their archaic modes of perception, even though the realistic ways of survival in the modern world have changed radically in terms of work and of society. And not recently, but many generations ago.

Awareness of the persistence of the two genetic types underneath the outward forms of modern society is highly relevant to the understanding of the psychobiological dynamics that led to the conditions responsible for the cancer epidemic. These two types together comprise the majority of the population. In the United States, diseases of the locomotor system ("rheumatism") are the most frequent form of chronic disease (Perrott, 1945), and half the population dies of some form of cardiovascular disease. The two types have one common characteristic: they are primarily "thing-oriented." Genetically, both are dominated by the psychobiological motivations that allowed their forebears to survive as conquerors of prehuman nature: the hunters killing and eventually domesticating animals more powerful than man; the planters clearing woods and grasslands from wild vegetation and replacing it with plants that support human existence. In the modern age, finally, the spirit of conquest proceeded to the point at which even human infants became "things." As we saw in the preceding chapter, however, this thing-orientation has had destructive consequences for the health of those children who are genetically dominated by the need to live a human-oriented life. In psychoanalytical terms, these subjects are dominated by the genital instinct, the striving for love and procreation.

Apparently the evolution and growth of the human species have, in the past, been due to the effectiveness of social forces that maintained a biological balance between the powers of the thing-oriented and of the human-oriented members of the various types of culture. The contemporary loss of this balance (cf. Chapter, V, p. 135 ff.) makes it important to consider the basic dynamics of the archaic thing-oriented cultures and the historical developments that allowed them to encroach upon the physiological use of the sexual and nursing functions.

Hunter societies can be traced back to Neanderthal Man, who flourished 30,000 years ago and has survived in various parts of the world until the present time. Campbell describes our European ancestors, who left an ample pictorial record of their lives in French and Spanish caves, as "an extraordinarily sturdy race...fighting it out in a landscape calling for every bit of wit and spunk at their disposal. Originally bow and arrow had not been invented...the chase was pursued with wooden, flint-pointed spears, while the animals sought and slain were the mammoth, rhinoceros, bison, brown bear and cave bear. These beasts were pursued afoot and met face to face, at close quarters."

The religions of hunting tribes are characterized by the belief in the individual immortality of the souls of man and animal. In their magic techniques, the bone, as the indestructible part of the body, plays an important role in controlling the spirits of the dead. A man's conviction of personal immortality minimizes his fear of death and also his fear of offending the spirit of the slain animal.

Leadership is exercised by shamans. They reveal their divine inspiration by their spontaneous initiative and by their capacity for going into trances. Identification with the hunted animals is part of their magic. Pictures of shamans wearing animal masks are found in the caves of Spain and France. In view of what follows later, it should be mentioned that hunters never practice ritual human sacrifice of members of their own tribe. Evidently they place a high value on the individual human being.

Although *contemporary culture* rarely provides scope for the hunter type of personality, the *dominance of locomotor intentionality* finds ways of expressing itself in the life style and disease liability of such individuals:

1. The *use of the locomotor system* in itself provides pleasurable experience. Because only a few individuals can find this satisfaction in their work, they often put excessive energy into the accomplishment of their tasks and into their sports. The nonsporting individuals just enjoy walking and often travel.

2. They *assert their individuality* in work and in social relationships. As children they identify themselves with the dominant parent, and as adults they pursue their idiosyncratic goals fearlessly in the face of great obstacles. Material conditions and the pressure of social convention certainly can be as formidable as the monsters their ancestors hunted.

3. When they don't succeed in accomplishing their aims, their locomotor system *expresses their individuality in the form of somatic symptoms:* when they become crippled by arthritis or Parkinsonism, their unwillingness to submit to external pressures becomes structural, they *cannot* bend; yet until the very end muscular tension plays a decisive part in the vicious circle of their disease processes. (For clinical illustrations I refer the interested reader to my pertinent publications: 1937b, 1939a, 1946a, 1946b, 1948).

Planter societies evolved much later than those of the hunters, about 9,000 years ago, and they have maintained their basic life style in many parts of the world until the present time. Like the hunters, their ancestors had been primitive food gatherers. But whereas following the free-moving, capricious game had appealed to individuals dominated by the needs of the locomotor system, the nature of plant life had appealed to individuals dominated by the needs of the cardiovascular system. Plants are rooted in the ground and survive by adjusting their growth to the seasonal rhythm of their environment. The cardiovascular system represents the evolution of the basic system by which the earliest forms of life survived in the oceans. Those depended passively on the nutrients their milieu provided. At most, they increased the flow of sea water by rhythmic motions to pump it through their hollow bodies. As evolution produced more complex bodies, the vital nutrient fluid was internalized and developed into blood, and its circulation became the task of the cardiovascular system. But these developments did not change the basic system's primordial character, the complete dependency on the environment and on those other organ systems that actively seek out and incorporate food and oxygen, and process the intake chemically until it can be carried by the blood stream to the individual cells of all the body organs.

The functional homology of plant life and the cardiovascular system explains that individuals in whom the latter dominated became particularly adept at organizing their life style in harmony with the behavior of the plants on which they depended. They settled near their fields and gardens. Individual inititative was subordinated to the seasonal stages of their plants, from seed to fruit. Women as the embodiment of fertility assumed greater social importance than in hunting societies, which depended on the year-round free mobility of men.

Planter societies had no use for the individualistic leadership of shamans, but were ordered by priests. Priests saw to it that the individual members religiously observed the all-important seasons of the year, and tried to influence the crops magically by the ritualistic order of community life, and by special celebrations of important days. There was a very practical reason for the fact that the priestly functions were exercised by men: Woman were at the beck and call of the infants on whose survival the community depended, whereas men were free to synchronize their religious observances with the set pace of the daily and seasonal movement of sun, moon, and stars.

In keeping with the collective character of planter societies, immortality, too, was collective. The individual human being was equated with the seed of the plant, which is buried and resurrected as a new plant. Priesthood and kingship were not acquired by personal charisma, but conferred by ritual order. Ego boundaries were periodically dissolved in collective ceremonies and orgies.

In the Old World and in the New, the subordination of the individual to the life of the community found its extreme expression in the institution of human sacrifice. To insure magically that the buried seed would bring a rich harvest, a select couple was ceremonially killed and buried after ritual intercourse. On the most primitive level of culture, it had to be a particularly healthy couple; on the higher levels it had to be the king and his consort or consorts. The sacrificial couple had to be worthy of enacting the death and resurrection of the spirits that controlled the fertility of the soil.

Contemporary culture obviously favors the breeding of individuals who are, like the prehistoric planters, genetically predisposed to conform to the demands of an impersonal provider of their survival needs. Language bears testimony to the archaic background of this social attitude, "plant" being used equally for real plants and for factories, by some ministers even for their parish buildings.

Children of the cardiovascular type usually identify themselves with the conforming parent, and as adults they conform to the social values of their environment.[9] The performance of their cardiovascular system depends on their self-perception as measuring up to their social image, to what their social environment has expected of them. Some die when they feel they have accomplished their mission in life; others, when they have lost all hope of ever accomplishing it. In still other instances, cardiovascular failures and recoveries reflect changing states of their social standing. President Eisenhower demonstrated this point most dramatically when he suffered a coronary attack in the midst of the controversy over whether he should seek a second term of office. The public reaction answered Eisenhower's doubts on the political and social level for many years to come. Then there are the many cases of slowly progressing cardiovascular and social deterioration in which the symptoms fluctuate impressively in parallel with the situation of the moment.

The preceding review of the survival of the prehistoric hunters and planters as distinct psychobiological types in our midst may seem strange. It is obvious that modern white populations are descendants of these prehistoric ancestors, but after thousands of years of mixed breeding one would have expected a greater variety of types. There are, however, two factors that favor these two most frequent (cf. p. 172) forms of clustering:

1. Capacity for taking individualistic action and capacity for adapting to the conventions of society have both, each in its own way, very high survival value and are likely to have been bred into dominant genetic qualities.
2. The family studies and the specific test of L. Szondi (1939, 1944, 1948, 1959) have demonstrated that many individuals are sexually drawn together by their unconscious genetic needs rather than by their conscious, often patently erroneous, impressions of each other. Independently of Szondi, Friedrich Curtius (1959) has found in the contemporary population families in which arthritis and Parkinsonism are prevalent, others in which cardiovascular diseases predominate.

VII

Biological Links Between Industrial Civilization and Cancer

"I personally have the feeling that the problem of cancer is not merely a biology and a laboratory problem. But it belongs to a certain extent to the realm of philosophy. This, an X in the pathology of cancer, is a principle we do not understand yet. While we can understand most pathological processes as defense reactions or as healing processes, here we are facing a fact that does not fit at all into our general biological conceptions."

—Henry Sigerist

A. Migration, Tuberculosis and Cancer

The most immediate and marked effect of the Industrial Revolution was an epidemic increase of tuberculosis. Infection by the mycobacterium tuberculosis had been endemic since antiquity, but the majority of the population had established peaceful coexistence with the microbe. This was consistent with the symbiotic relationship between man and his natural environment that prevailed when the majority of the population cultivated the soil. Bacteria are part of the natural environment. Dubos (1965) has analyzed in detail how, under conditions of unusual stress, the equilibrium between the human organism and certain bacteria breaks down in the genetically susceptible part of the population.

Unusual stress was brought to bear on the masses of the population whom the Industrial Revolution forced to migrate from the country into factory towns and city slums. Whereas tuberculosis remained rare in the countryside, it became the most frequent cause of death, the "white plague," in the cities (Dubos & Dubos, 1952).

There were at least three factors that contributed to the high mortality rate of the tuberculosis-prone population:

1. The working classes were forced to subsist on starvation diets. It is an established fact that "*nutritional deficiencies* play a decisive role in the prevalence and severity of microbial diseases among underprivileged people" (Dubos, 1965).

2. The stressful living conditions activated the mycobacteria that everybody carried by way of raising the *cortisone production* (Dubos, 1965).

3. Tuberculosis-prone personalities are characterized by their tendency to become deeply attached to their families. They were particularly traumatized by the *separations enforced by survival needs*. Kissen (1958) studied this aspect of the problem very thoroughly in immigrant populations. His findings are supported by the Rorschach findings (Chapter III): that tuberculosis patients are characterized by exceptional need for affection.

Since 1850 the incidence of tuberculosis has steadily declined, but there has been a complementary rise in cancer deaths. This phenomenon, first discovered by Sir Thomas Coglan in 1902, was thoroughly substantiated by Cherry (1924, 1925) and confirmed by Berkson in 1960. Cherry found that since 1850 the *combined number of adult deaths from tuberculosis and cancer* in Australia, Europe, New Zealand and North America accounted for 20 percent of the yearly total of deaths in these countries. That this ratio has remained stable for more than a century leads to the conclusion that tuberculosis and cancer are alternate disease liabilities of a genetic subgroup of Caucasian populations.

The hypothesis of a genetic link between the two diseases finds support in clinical experience. I mentioned earlier that not infrequently cancer patients had been tuberculous earlier in life. This sequence has been reported most frequently for localization in the lungs (Westergren, 1959; Schwartz, 1960) and in the skin (Schwartz, 1960). Usually the association has been interpreted as causal: that the tissue damage of tuberculosis provides the soil favoring cancerous proliferation. The report of Collas (1964) from a tuberculosis sanatorium, however, indicates that of the 30 cancers observed in a five-year period, 13 developed in organs not involved in the tubercular process; furthermore, that the tubercular process became inactive at the time at which the cancer appeared. This was contrary to the clinical expectation that the cancer cachexia would aggravate the tuberculosis. Collas therefore considered the possibility that both diseases have a common genetic background. Other evidence has been provided by Warthin (1913), who obtained detailed family histories of 30 cancer patients, covering two to three generations. Not infrequently he found a tuberculosis ancestry in patients without cancer in the preceding generations. Recently, Salk (1969) and Weiss (1969) have demonstrated that in mice and monkeys certain immunological relationships exist between tuberculosis and cancer.

As long as one considered only the great differences of the somatic processes and of the personality type, the close relationship between tuberculosis and cancer remained mysterious. Nevertheless, there is *one common factor*: Tuberculosis and cancer patients depend upon *intense object relationships*, and their illnesses consist in the creation of internal substitutes for lost external objects.

The *difference* between the two diseases was defined in terms of psychosexual development: Tuberculosis patients are primarily genital characters; cancer patients are largely fixated on the pregenital, anal level. Since the rise of cancer is taking place within the same genetic group, the progressive change suggests that an exogenous agent has conditioned the shift from genital to pregenital object relationships.

B.   The Effect of Depersonalized Nursing

An agent capable of producing the observed psychosexual effects must fulfill three conditions:

1. Exposure to the agent takes place in the first year of life, when the infantile organism is plastic enough to be transformed biologically by exogenous influences.
2. The agent began to become influential in the beginning of the 19th century, because the rapid increase in cancer deaths began at the time when those born in the beginning of the century had reached cancer age.
3. The influence of the agent must have been spreading and affecting an ever-increasing number of genetically tuberculosis-prone individuals.

There is only one new factor which answers to this description:

The change from breast-feeding to artificial feeding.

Artificial feeding began with the economic pressures of the Industrial Revolution on women who became mothers. They were forced to return to the factory at the earliest possible moment after having given birth. Their babies had to be "dry-fed" by grandmothers, maiden aunts, and older siblings. In the first half of the 19th century, only few babies survived; but gradually the methods of artificial feeding became more effective. In 1845 Elijah Pratt (Drake, 1948) invented the rubber nipple, in 1860 Liebig (Sunley, 1955) developed the first good formula, and in 1886 Von Soxleth introduced a practical apparatus for pasteurizing the daily milk rations in individual bottles.

Statisticians have shown remarkably little interest in the extent and success of artificial feeding. I found only the report of the city of Berlin for 1886. In that year, 68 *percent* of all newborn babies were bottle-fed, and 41 percent of them survived the first year of life. It may be assumed that these figures reflect the prevailing situation in the *industrialized* and *urban* communities of that period in other countries of the Western world. These communities are known to have contributed specifically to the rise of tuberculosis (Dubos, 1952) and of cancer (U.S. Pub. Health Serv., 1964).

In the last decade of the 19th century, medical textbooks agree (Bruening, 1908; Brenneman, 1942) artificial feeding became increasingly effective insofar as *physical survival* was concerned. Medical science provided the techniques for providing industrial society with the needed numbers of workers and consumers. In the Twenties of the present century, many physicians became convinced that artificial feeding was as healthy as breast-feeding. This climate of opinion is reflected specifically in the fact that the mothers of the upper socio-economic classes, frequently since antiquity unwilling to nurse their own babies, no longer used wet-nurses (Peiper, 1955).

Contentment with the survival rates of bottle-fed babies has been disturbed since the Forties by a growing concern with the psychobiological effects of artificial feeding. This concern had been voiced throughout the years by some physicians, but it was scientifically substantiated in 1945 when Spitz published his classic study of "hospitalism." Spitz demonstrated that, in the absence of an adequate amount of affectionate contact between baby and nurse, even perfect hygienic conditions are lethal for the very young and do lasting damage to the physical and psychological development of somewhat older children. Twelve years later (1957) Spitz warned "the thoughtful": "We may well wonder how extensively feeding babies a formula from a propped bottle may have influenced the development of the Western mind in the last 50 to 80 years. That such influence can be demonstrated in individual development is a matter of record. But the more important question arises, how this may have influenced changes in the ways of Western man, in the ways of his communication, and whether and how it has influenced his relations with his environment, his verbal and nonverbal symbols, and perhaps also his thinking processes."

The "propped bottle" is the extreme example of the mechanistic tendencies that have dominated the theories and, often, the practice of infant care in the industrialized world. These tendencies were the result of the new scientific approach to life as a purely biochemical process. Infants, in particular, were considered to have no needs other than physical: food, protection against cold and infection, and sleep. Consequently, physical contact between mother and baby tended to be limited to the physically necessary. For instance, tubes were introduced in 1864 to connect nipple and baby, a device that was modified and patented in 1910 as an "anti-embarrassment device." It allowed mothers who wanted to breast-feed their babies to do so without undressing. The accompanying picture shows a prim lady with the baby sprawling across her knees, holding the nipple to its mouth, as detached as a gas-station attendant. Between 1887 and 1945, the U.S. Patent Office granted nine patents for methods of propping up bottles (Drake, 1948). "Needless to say, even in those meager years, quite a few mothers continued to love their children 'against doctor's advice'—and we can congratulate them and their children for this. Fondling and cuddling one's child could not be suppressed." (Spitz, 1965)

Until 1942, the pamphlet "Infant Care" issued by the U.S. Children's Bureau subscribed to the mechanistic concept. The Bureau then revised it so much that Spitz found it "practically human," but he also noted the continued emphasis on physical needs. The new recommendation of demand feeding led to the result that the baby was always fed when it cried. Thus babies were often overfed when they actually had wanted to be played with.

Spitz made it clear that the issue in the first year of life is not the choice of nursing method, but the baby's *need for a minimum of physical affection*. Although such a minimum is provided by breast-feeding *nearly* automatically, this is not the case with mothers who do it in deference to external authority or to some intellectual or moral principle. Such mothers can breast-feed their babies so mechanically that the effect is apt to be more traumatic than relaxed bottle-feeding. The importance of a *genuine maternal attitude* in breast-feeding was clearly recognized by Sir William Cadogan (Ruhräh, 1925) in 1796, when he discussed the psychological problems of finding good wet-nurses. In the light of the preceding considerations, it is more appropriate to describe the new environmental factor accounting for the rise of cancer as *"depersonalized nursing,"* not as "bottle-feeding." The technique of feeding is only one of the media through which mothers can communicate affection to their babies.

When depersonalized nursing became popular, the *genetically tuberculosis-prone segment of the population was selectively vulnerable* to this practice. Many modern investigators (e.g., Antonelli and Seccia, 1956; Kissen, 1958; Wittkower, 1949) have confirmed the old observations that tuberculosis patients are characterized by "an inordinate need for affection." If this need is satisfied in the first year of life, the infants develop the capacity for easy relationships with their environment. Since antiquity, tuberculosis patients have been characterized by their nearly indestructible confidence that they will find eventually new love and new health even when they are forsaken and desperately sick. The famous "spes phthsica" is an exaggeration of the "basic trust" which Erikson (1963) described as the mark of an adequate relationship between baby and mother.

If, however, the "inordinate need for affection" is not satisfied in the first year of life, they do not trust that the world is going to provide replacements for lost objects of affection. The experience of limited options in the environment causes them to cling desperately to what they found (LeShan and Worthington, 1956) and become depressed if they lose a vital object.

The intense affectional needs of the tuberculosis/cancer genotype are different from the more numerous genotypes of the cardiovascular and the locomotor groups. These two clinical groups are characterized by the dominant need for fulfilling specific ego needs for which people and objects serve as mere implements. The cardiovascular group is primarily anxious for conformity with the social group (cf. Friedman's "type A," 1974; and Hinkle, 1968), the locomotor group is primarily concerned with acting according to their individualistic image. Certainly, all infants need a minimum of affection for survival, but the tuberculosis/cancer genotype has a lower frustration tolerance than other constitutional types.

C. *The Progressive Depersonalization of Human Relationships*

In the course of the last three decades, the great value of breast-

feeding has been widely acknowledged in scientific and popular literature. Nevertheless, physiological mothering has continued to decline
all over the world. Only in the college-educated upper middle classes
has breast-feeding become more popular. Newton and Newton (1967)
made the point that "lactation" is not an autonomous organ function,
but must be understood in the context of the psychological attitudes of
parents and of the medical profession. The authors provide conclusive
proof that, in spite of all evidence favoring breast-feeding, psychological resistance is spreading in the population and discouraging many
physicians from trying to influence their patients.

The cause of this psychological resistance has been clarified by the
work of Harlow (1965) on the development of affectional behavior in
monkeys. Paradoxically, Harlow's findings received a great deal of
publicity, but there has been general reluctance to apply them to the
contemporary human situation. Certainly, human beings and other
primates cannot be equated; but mothering does involve identifiable
biological elements that can be observed in experimental animals.

Radically depersonalized raising of rhesus monkeys on dummy
mothers established the fact that the method is superior to physiological nursing insofar as survival and physical health are concerned.
There are, however, serious consequences, if as babies they are raised
in isolation:

1. As adults, both males and females are *sexually incompetent.*
   In spite of normal sexual reactions to each other, they
   cannot copulate because they cannot coordinate their sexual
   reflexes.

2. The females which are impregnated on the "rape rack"
   become *"unnatural" mothers.* Without artificial feeding, all
   their first-born babies would die because the mothers fight
   them off savagely when they try to reach the nipples. Only
   those dummy-raised females who have second and third
   babies never become brutal, and generally fulfill the maternal
   role adequately, or even become *overprotective* (Seay, et al,
   1964).

3. The *first-born infants* of dummy-raised mothers, in playing
   with their peers, compensate for their deficient mothering
   by becoming *more orally active and sexually precocious*
   compared to their normally raised playmates (Seay, et al,
   1964).

These observations add up to the conclusion that the effects of
artificial nursing on subsequent generations are cumulative, the babies

becoming sexually inadequate, and their babies, in turn, becoming dependent on artificial feeding, thus carrying the disturbance from generation to generation to generation.

The parallels in the present bottle-fed human population are clear:

1. There is widespread *sexual incompetence*. This is evident from the great demand for sex education, books on sexual techniques, sexual exhibitionism, homosexuality, etc. Whereas throughout most of human history society tried to impose limitations on the tendency toward spontaneous heterosexual activity, the present mid-century is characterized by the paradoxical combination of heterosexual freedom and inability to enjoy the physiological act.

2. *Unnatural human mothers* have become more frequent. The "battered child syndrome" (Helfer and Kempe, 1968) has received a great deal of medical and legal attention; but these dreadful cases constitute the extreme of a phenomenon that is all too frequent: mothers who do not trust, or don't have spontaneous instincts, and turn to books for technical instruction.

3. *Compulsive oral activity and sexual precociousness* are much in evidence, specifically the rise of cigarette smoking, which will be discussed later.

All these parallels indicate that depersonalized nursing has profound and lasting biological effects that are not easily influenced by intellectual insight and conscious techniques. The decisive factor for the development of spontaneous affectionate interaction in nursing and in sexual intercourse is the early infantile experience of *the body of the mother*, not of the breast only. Harlow demonstrated that dummy-raised monkeys develop normal mating and mothering behavior if they are allowed to play with their peers. Thus, the milk bottle would not create problems if it were administered by women with natural instincts for affectionate behavior.

VIII

The Localization of Cancer

A. The Specificity of Functional Frustration

In the preceding chapters a wide variety of cancer sites provided material which demonstrated what all these patients had in common:
1. functional predominance of the anal over the genital type of object relationships;
2. biological and cultural conditioning which favors the development of the cancer-prone personality;
3. the loss of control over an object relationship which was vitally important to the patient.

The formulation "vitally important to the patient" needs to be qualified in this context, because it must be understood in terms of *personality needs*, not in terms of physical survival. It has been pointed out that life depends on complex symbiotic and social relationships and that death and disease can be brought on by their loss, most dramatically in the case of the so-called Voodoo deaths (Richter, 1959). Personality needs vary according to the genetic make-up of the given individual, which accounts for the fact that the *genetically dominant needs are apt to be most sensitive to frustration.* As a consequence, the organ carrying the dominant function is most likely to become sick. In the case of the cancer-prone personality it is to be expected that the *lost external object will be internalized as a neoplastic tumor of the organ carrying the frustrated dominant function.*

The preceding hypothesis can be validated in several forms of cancer. The data on the association between organ site and specific environmental frustrations have been collected by independent observers, in all cases without any awareness that the statistical findings had social and psychological implications.

Stomach cancer, for instance, has been found to be associated frequently with poverty (U.S. Pub. Health Serv., 1964). Among the industrialized nations its highest incidence occurs in Japan; the lowest, in the United States. That this discrepancy is not due to a genetic difference of the populations can be concluded from the fact that stomach cancer in the United States was twice as frequent in 1930 as in 1960. During this period the gene pool did not change, but the level of prosperity certainly did. At the same time there is a genetic factor involved since the disease occurs only in a small segment of the population afflicted by the experience of an empty stomach. It apparently depends also on the personality type, the degree an individual suffers from deprivation in this form. In tuberculosis, another frequent disease of the poor, the patients appear to be affected indirectly, by the emotional deprivation entailed by devitalization.

It is unlikely that the factor causing stomach cancer is the direct effect of physical undernourishment. Observations on the stomach ulcer by Mittelman, Wolff and Sharp (1942) have shown that in this form of stomach disease the patients are *specifically sensitive to the experience of being deprived of psychological sustenance.* Thus stomach cancer occurs also among those who are well-fed physically, particularly those who overeat because they feel starved emotionally. The portly figure of Pope John XXIII provides a historical example. His personal strength had been fed by the world-embracing charity of the Mother Church. Trusting his own experience and his unique position he conceived the idea of the Vatican Council as the means to make this ecumenical good will available to those outside of the Church. With the single-minded determination of the cancer-prone personality he pursued this goal until he found himself fatally deprived of the expected and needed support from his own Curia. When he realized that the original object of his labors was lost through this form of starvation, the internalized object in the form of stomach cancer became the end of his life.

The receptive side of the oral function predominates in stomach cancer, but *breast cancer* is characterized by the need to give. Numerous studies have confirmed that the more fully women have used their breasts in nursing babies, the less liable they are to develop this form of cancer. As in all diseases the liability is a product of genetic predisposition and of intensity of frustration. As Bagg (1936) demonstrated, breast cancer occurs in 15 percent of mice genetically not cancer-prone, if the litter is removed immediately after birth. Since the majority of modern women subject themselves to the same experience as Bagg's mice, it is apparent that for many of them this frustration is not important enough to cause cancer.

Another difficulty in ascertaining the nature of an irretrievable loss preceding cancer occurs in those cases where only the *nature of the relationship is changed.* A naive observer might assume that the change would have satisfied the patient. For example, I know several cases of breast cancer in very superior women after their husbands had unexpectedly achieved economic or intellectual independence. One very striking example has been described by Anton Boisen (1960) in great detail without any awareness of the psychodynamics. After his schizophrenic episode he had felt a "wretch in need of the compassion" of Alice Batchelder, a remarkable friend during 25 years of an asexual relationship. She developed a fatal breast cancer at the time when his classic *Exploration of the Inner World* (1935) was going to press. As the dedication acknowledges, the fact that he could "depend on her unswerving fidelity" made the book possible. It must have been obvious to Alice Batchelder that he had achieved independence from his spiritual mother.

As in stomach cancer, the problem of frustration in breast cancer is complicated by psychological factors. Smalheiser and Tarlau (1951) as well as Bacon, Renneker and Cutler (1952) observed that breast cancer patients are frequently characterized by poorly integrated genital behavior which can even preclude the possibility of biological motherhood. At the same time their behavior shows a possessive attitude toward their physical or adopted children and furthermore an overflowing of "the milk of human kindness," often to the extent that they are incapable of expressing hostility. Both research teams found evidence that this psychological constellation is rooted in unresolved hostility toward their own mothers and is then overcompensated through compulsive, often masochistic solicitude for others. All this can be summarized in one sentence. The dominant function in breast-cancer-prone women is the need to nurse others physically or socially, although satisfaction is inhibited by hostile and possessive feelings regarding the recipient of this care. This conclusion is substantiated in greater detail by the psychoanalytical study of five breast cancer patients by Renneker and his co-workers (1963).

The breast cancer group bears close resemblance to the results of mechanical feeding in rhesus monkeys: females deprived of normal mothering became sexually incompetent, and, if they could be forced into child-bearing and nursing, they became possessive mothers (cf. Chapter V). In human females, bottle-feeding leads to the same results, except for the modifications due to their greater psychological freedom. The experience of sexual incompetence leads easily to an attitude of avoidance. Nursing is not induced by an instinctual mechanism but by a sense of duty and takes the form of substitute behavior, e.g., the choice of a profession in caring for children, the physically ill and for the economically deprived, or the manner in which authority is exercised.

The two group studies quoted above were confirmed by Wheeler and Caldwell (1955) with respect to the essential conclusions of their predecessors. It is inherent in the nature of group studies that the need for abstractions, the complexity of human individualities and the critical bias of later investigators entail also some divergencies with respect to details. Case histories published without a general thesis, but in adequate clinical detail, are apt to convey more convincingly the specific dynamics which characterize breast cancer. Earlier I referred to the case of Alice Batchelder which Anton Boisen published, unintentionally as far as psychosomatic conclusions were concerned. Inman (1961) revealed the life history of a maternity nurse which illustrates in detail all the points made in this monograph in respect of the development of the cancer-prone personality, breast localization and the social factor in the course of the neoplastic process.[10]

Breast cancer provides a good example for *the importance of psychodynamic considerations in cancer prophylaxis*. Statistics (Adair and Bagg, 1925; MacDonald, 1942; Quisenberry, 1960; Marcial, 1960) have demonstrated that breast cancer is a specific hazard in populations where women do not nurse their children. If the physical act alone were important, deliberate breast-feeding would go a long way toward reducing this form of cancer. The preceding psychological observations, however, indicate that genetically predisposed women are likely to have been traumatized by their own infantile nursing experiences. The familial incidence of breast cancer is known to be high (Hoernecke and Berndt, 1965). Such women, therefore, are apt to be poorly motivated for having babies and for nursing them without ambivalence. Breast-feeding as a purely hygienic, self-protective or moralistic act entails emotional conflict and the risk of recreating mother hostility in the next generation. There is, therefore, a certain danger in the otherwise welcome reawakening interest in breast-feeding. Possibly less hostility is generated if the mother does not try to fight a spontaneous aversion to this act (Bruch, 1952; Borstelmann, 1965). Allowing women to *choose* motherhood and the form of nursing according to their own feelings permits the *self-limiting potential of breast cancer dynamics* to take effect in place of the current self-perpetuating trend. Once the damage of a frustrating nursing experience has been inflicted on a breast-cancer-prone woman, the resulting antisexual and antinursing disposition would result automatically in the reduction of the hereditary risk in the population and particularly its secondary psychobiological consequences.

Cervix cancer is the liability of a personality type which presents a clear contrast to the breast cancer group. Motivation for genital activity predominates over the interest in a nursing, possessive relationship with others. The evidence for the role of genital frustration is negative as well as positive.

The negative evidence is that this localization for cancer is rare in virgins and practically non-existent in nuns (Gagnon, 1950; Stephenson and Grace, 1954; Towne, 1955) although not all nuns are virgins—some have even raised children before turning to religious life. The choice of monastic life, however, appears to be reliable evidence for a *very limited interest in sexual self-expression*. At first sight one might consider convent life incompatible with the cancer-prone personality because the vows of obedience and poverty conflict with the predominant striving for individualistic object control. Actually, however, the convent often provides the social setting for this need, either in the mode of religious pursuit, or in the orders devoted to nursing and teaching. Cancer of the uterus, for instance, is six times more frequent in nuns than in the general population. This is confirmed by the same study which established the rarity of cervix cancer in nuns (Gagnon, 1950).

Positive evidence for the strong genital motivation of this group is provided by numerous studies (Tarlau and Smalheiser, 1951; Stephenson and Grace, 1954; Pereyra, 1961; Christopherson and Parker, 1965), which establish that cervical cancer is found with particular frequency in women who begin to have intercourse before the age of twenty, and pursue an active sex life in an autistic fashion as is implied by their high divorce rate and promiscuity. This way of life is particularly significant because it is pursued so frequently in spite of frustration as far as satisfaction is concerned. Stephenson and Grace (1954), for example, found that failure to reach orgasm occurred twice as often in this group as in women with cancer of other organs. This means that the general difficulty for the cancer-prone to experience orgasms is particularly frustrating for women who are highly motivated and experienced (see Chapter III, Plate VI). They are therefore likely to develop invasive cancer when they have lost hope. Rotkin (1962) observed that cervix cancer develops after a mean period of thirty years after the beginning of sexual relationships. This is obviously the time of life when many sexually frustrated women experience "curfew panic" and give up hope, the typical cancerogenic situation.

Rotkin tried to explain the beginning sexual activity and the onset of cancer thirty years later by a number of assumptions derived from Auster's discovery (1965) that smegma contains a cancerogenic virus, an explanation for the fact that cervical cancer is extremely rare in Jewish women. Rotkin assumed that before the age of twenty the cervix is more vulnerable than later on, that the smegma virus creates, therefore, more frequently a precancerous lesion which has a mean latency period of thirty years. These arbitrary hypotheses do not explain why these patients have greater sexual need than the general population. He also failed to consider this personality trait as the reason for the early beginning of intercourse and of the frequent onset of cancer in the late forties.

In Rotkin's psychological study (Rotkin, et al, 1965), he did not indicate whether he had changed the *prophylactic recommendations* he suggested in 1962 on the basis of his somatic theory: postponement of sexual intercourse until after the age of twenty and frequent Papanicoloau tests for impatient teenagers. If one considers the role of personality in the genesis of cervix cancer, his recommendations would seem to increase rather than decrease the risk. They are liable to create additional complications in the sex life of a woman who starts with the handicap of an anal personality orientation, which makes satisfaction of her strong genital needs difficult. The fewer hypochondriacal and moralistic feelings are associated with the sexual act, the more likely it is that the conflict may be outgrown and cancerogenic frustration avoided.

In the male sex, cancer of the *prostate gland* results from a similar conflict between genital activity and inadequate satisfaction. Epidemiological studies (Quisenberry, 1960; Marcial, 1960) indicate that this neoplastic site prevails in cultures where men often engage in lovemaking stopped short of coitus. This conclusion is supported by microscopic studies of prostate glands. Franks (1954, 1956) found that *precancerous* cell changes increase steadily from 4 percent in the age group 40-49 to 83 percent in the age group beyond 90. The incidence of *invasive cancer*, however, increased only up to the age of 80, from 5 percent before the age of 50, to 40 percent in the age group between 70 and 79; then decreases to 5 percent at the age of 80 and above. Flocks (1965) in a study of 4,000 cases confirmed the rising frequency up to the age of 80 and the subsequent decrease of invasive cancer. He also made the point that with increasing age the life expectancy of prostatic cancer patients rises consistently.

The age of 80 as a dividing point between increasing and decreasing incidence and malignancy of prostate cancer corresponds to Kinsey's findings (1948) that at that age complete impotence occurs in nearly 100 percent of the male population. This means that with the end of sexual arousal, experiences of sexual frustration are reduced. Thus, in spite of the greater frequency of cancer *in situ* after 80, the intensity of sexual frustration is lessened to such an extent that the change to invasiveness occurs much more rarely. Epidemiology, histology and sexology support statistically the conclusion that the localization of cancer in the prostate gland is the male analogon to cervix cancer. Pathogenesis is the result of the frustration inherent in the combination of the anal type of object relationship with a high motivation for genital activity. *In both sexes cancer in situ seems to be the somatic expression of the psychological condition in which these patients spent their lives while they were in good physical health.* As LeShan and Worthington (1956) found, they had suffered deep emotional frustration early in life, but endeavored to compensate for it painfully, until an irretrievable loss robbed them of all hope that they could maintain the former minimum of satisfaction.

The preceding four examples of cancer localization substantiate the clinical correctness of Freud's (1920) formulation of the *death instinct* as the striving of every organism to safeguard its own individual path toward death. This individual path is characterized by two identifiable constitutional factors:

1. the predominance of the anal type of object relationships;
2. the predominance of the psychobiological values
   of a specific organ function.

The combination of both factors accounts for the specific quality of the precancerous personality development and for the eventual production of the tumor in the organ which had played the leading part. Unless therapeutic intervention succeeds in changing the psychodynamic situation (Chapter IX) the neoplasia ends in death. Since the tumor site is isomorphic with the life pattern the organism succeeds indeed in safeguarding the individual path toward death to the very end.

When Freud described this overall behavior of organisms as death *instinct* his intuition went far ahead of his contemporaries and of his own scientific knowledge. In his time instincts were considered to be aimed directly at the objects which are necessary for the self-preservation of the individual and for the survival of the species. They served "life" and the concept of a "death instinct" was therefore a self-contradictory term. Freud recognized this and tried to justify the paradox by pointing to the irrational character of instincts and by relegating the death instinct to the unconscious as the silent antagonist of the "noisy" life instinct.

Today Freud would not have encountered any difficulties in conceptualizing his clinical observations as instinctual behavior. Tinbergen (1955) concluded from many careful experiments on animals that the end of purposive behavior is not the attainment of an object or a situation for itself, but *the performance of the consummatory action.* "Not the litter or the food is the animal striving towards, but the performance itself of the maternal activities or eating." Under normal environmental conditions these performances sustain life because organisms are usually born into situations which contain the vital objects to which the instincts are attuned. It can be demonstrated, however, by dummies, that animals persevere in their instinctual behavior even though it entails frustration and death. Life and death are both secondary results of innate behavior patterns just as litters are raised as by-products of maternal behavior, not because the females *intend* these results. It is the primary character of life to create forms, not only of the body, but also of behavior. The latter, as Lorenz pointed out, is often more useful for taxonomic purposes than the dissection of the corpses.

In the light of modern biological knowledge the only antiquated part of Freud's definition of the death instinct is its teleological phrasing. Neither life nor death as such can be pursued. They are both mere abstractions from the concrete events in which "life" and "death" take place. When Freud objectified these abstractions as specific instincts, as the war between the mythological powers of Eros and Thanatos, he acted like the "learned exponents of Einstein" whom Whitehead (1920) chided at that time for their failure to realize that "space," "time" and "electron" do not exist as separate realities in addition to the space-time continuum in which they are observed. Whitehead likened the irrationality of objectified abstractions to the smile which the Cheshire cat abstracts from its body in "Alice in Wonderland."

Divested of its poetic dramatization, "death instinct" simply sums up the behavior of all organisms, whether protozoa or homo sapiens.

As Rorschach's 10 dummies of existential situations demonstrate (p. 33ff, Chapters II and III), even the most intelligent individual perceives the objective environment only within the limitations of his constitutional potential and can only react accordingly. Thus animal and man proceed from conception to death by behaving according to the specific instinctual equipment. Since instincts are purposeful under average natural conditions, organisms are bound to give the appearance of "striving" to safeguard their individual paths towards death. Actually, life lasts as long as the innate instinctual equipment is supported by innate vitality and by satisfactory environmental conditions. The relative strength of the various instincts accounts for the congruity between life history and form of death. The end comes when vitality is exhausted or the environment fails to provide for satisfaction of vital needs.

Obviously there is interdependence between the internal and external factors. When young people meet with seemingly hopeless external frustration their greater vitality becomes invested in the more rapid growth of the tumor as the internalized object, whereas the waning vitality of older people causes usually a gradual loss of effective contact with vital objects and a slower replacement by the tumor.

The preceding analysis of specific forms of cancer is given because they illustrate rather plainly the dynamics of localized neoplasia. In the case of lung cancer a more complex problem presents itself.

B. Lung Cancer

1. The Psychological Role of the Lungs

Tokuhata and Lilienfeld (1963) demonstrated that lung cancer involves two independent genetic variables:
    a. predisposition for the neoplastic process in general; and
    b. predisposition for the *localization* of the process in
       the lungs.[11]

The latter variable links lung cancer with other disease processes of the respiratory system, such as tuberculosis, asthma bronchiale, and emphysema. It appears therefore likely that the common genetic factor is responsible not only for the disease liability of the organ, but also for *the functional dominance of a related component of psychobiological dynamics.* The nature of this personality component is suggested by the implications of two epidemiological facts which have been established for tuberculosis and cancerous lung disease alike. They are:

a. the highest incidence occurs in the *lowest income* groups (Dubos, 1952; U.S. Pub. Health Serv., 1964).

b. the mortality is increased among *migrants*.

With respect to mortality, it has been observed that in tuberculosis (Dubos, 1952; Kissen, 1958) and in lung cancer (U.S. Pub. Health Serv., 1964) it has been higher among those who had moved from rural into urban districts than among those born in the latter. In the case of lung cancer, this applies equally to smokers and nonsmokers (U.S. Pub., Health Serv., 1964). Immigration into foreign countries has also entailed higher mortality due to tuberculosis (Kissen, 1958) and to lung cancer (Eastcott, 1956; Dean, 1959). This is true in lung cancer even though the new country may be as little afflicted with air pollution as agricultural New Zealand (Eastcott, 1956).

The association of two heterogeneous lung diseases with migration suggests that *the respiratory function is related to the potential for freedom from the given environment.* Whatever the specific motivations for leaving the native milieu may be, the decision to do so requires a greater spirit of independence than to stay put, except in cases of extreme economic or political pressures. A suggested interpretation is that migrant populations are likely to include a higher than average percentage of individuals in whom the psycho-biological influence of the lungs is particularly strong due to the genetic factor mentioned above.

The concept of the respiratory function as expression of need for independence is supported by the fact that the two diseases are most frequent in the *lowest income* groups. They are obviously most handicapped in the exercise of a desire for freedom and therefore reduced to somatic self-expression.

The preceding inferences from epidemiology are in keeping with more general considerations.

In the course of *evolution* it was the development of the lungs which enabled animal life to abandon its original aquatic habitat and to find living space on land and in the air. The emigration of organisms from the water was the crucial step which led to the emergence of man, to his supreme freedom of choosing his habitat anywhere on earth.

In *ontogenesis* every human being still repeats this original phylogenetic event. The first breath still marks the moment when the individual emerges from the amniotic fluid and becomes independent from the maternal bloodstream. Everybody, no matter how old, continues to respond with a deep breath to the experience of liberation from a physically or psychologically confining situation.

In the sphere of pathology "the first breath" is reenacted dramatically in *bronchial asthma*. French and Alexander (1941) found that the attack is elicited by an acute conflict between striving for independence and awareness of dependent needs. Incapable of resolving the impasse realistically, the patient expresses his situation symbolically by filling his lungs compulsively with air. At the same time the distressing condition expresses a reaching out for a supportive mother or mother-substitute. This experience is characteristically most frequent during the developmental years; it becomes rarer later on. Most asthmatics achieve a realistic balance between their independency needs and their capacity for living on their individual level of "aspiration." Those who fail in this endeavor are apt to develop emphysema. The substance of the organ of freedom diminishes, and the space is filled with air, the original object. I am aware that some authors have objected to the preceding concept of French and Alexander that it is not "scientifically validated" (Purcell, 1965), but I have never encountered a clinical case yet which differed from their psychodynamic model.

In the case of *tuberculosis* the object of independent reaching out is of a symbiotic nature. This has been discussed at length in the analysis of the Rorschach responses which prevail in this group (Chapter III). It appeared that the mycobacterium tuberculosis, not so long ago nearly as freely available as the air, became pathogenic when human partnership failed because of direct emotional frustration, or because devitalization made symbiotic life impossible. Tuberculosis was the most frequent cause of death in the period of industrialization when the masses where subjected to minimal wages and their individual freedom restricted by harsh labor conditions and mechanized factory work. At the same time the strictures of Victorian morality filled the poor with guilt, not only about actions but even about their carnal desires (Thompson, 1964). The frequency of tuberculosis among immigrants is generally lower than in their countries of origin because for some the migration provides the opportunity to satisfy the vital needs which had motivated them. There is, however, one significant exception which was pointed out by Kissen (1958). In 1931 the incidence of tuberculosis was 130 per 100,000 of the population in Ireland, and 140 among the Irish immigrants in the U.S.A. Kissen explains this phenomenon as the result of the particularly strong bond of the Irish for the home country. Their motive for leaving is therefore chiefly unbearable economic pressure, not striving for independence, although without some ingredient of the latter the immigrants would have accepted starvation at home. Apparently, for the Irish immigrants the trauma of separation from country and family was frequently so damaging that the economic advantages of the new country could not compensate for it. Thus, the Irish illustrate the association between tuberculosis and symbiotic needs.

2. Epidemiology of Lung Cancer

The lung-cancer-prone personality is characterized by the combined effects of two constitutionally dominant needs:

a. the genetic *predisposition of the lungs* determines specific striving for independence from the given environment.

b) the genetic and constitutional *predisposition for cancer* determines specific striving for control over the chosen objects in accordance with the anal fixation of the personality type.

The neoplastic process develops when the pursuit of these needs meets with apparently hopeless frustration. As pointed out above, low income and immigrant status entail a higher risk of disease. This is plausible because low income puts the lung cancer personality at a greater disadvantage than those who find satisfaction in "making ends meet" wherever they have been placed by fate. Migrants are apt to find their social and economic goals restricted by the natives, if not by xenophobia, at least by their greater familiarity with the opportunities for getting ahead. This interpretation of the higher disease incidence among *immigrants* is also supported by the fact that they have a lower incidence than the population from which they originated. Their intermediate position between the mortality rates of the old and the new country, respectively, suggests that in spite of the difficulties mentioned, a significant number of immigrants succeed in finding what they had been looking for. This is consistent with the individualistic orientation of the cancer group (Eastcott, 1956; Dean, 1959, 1961, 1962).

The great variations of the lung cancer mortality from country to country provided further illustrations for the psychodynamics of this disease. The following examples, excepting the figures for Japan (Todd, 1959), are taken from the tabulation of Doll (1955) which intended to demonstrate that the variations of cigarette consumption are "not inconsistent" with a causal relationship to the incidence of lung cancer. Since this ratio (0.73 ± 0.30) is not very impressive, it is interesting to point out the psychosocial aspects of his findings (Fig. 2).

Great Britain has by far the highest rate of all countries. Its history proves that in the course of the last 350 years the British people have produced the greatest number of individuals motivated for migration and capable of controlling the countries in which they settled. Presently this population is hemmed in by the fact that the world is no longer as open for emigration as in the centuries of the expanding Empire. At home the population density is second only to that of Holland. Since the genetic stock has not been changed by large-scale immigration, the conclusion may be drawn that the population of Great Britain includes a particularly high share of lung cancer personalities who are subjected to specifically frustrating socio-economic conditions. This explanation is supported by the fact that in the three former colonies, *Australia, Canada* and the *United States* the lung cancer rate is less than half of that of Great Britain. Australia, which is settled nearly exclusively by British immigrants, and is also one of the most highly urbanized countries, may serve as a good example for the concept that successful emigration reduces the hazard of lung cancer. As noted above (p. 184) the representation of lung cancer personalities is likely to be higher among the immigrants than among those who stayed at home.

Holland has only 53 percent of the lung cancer rate of Great Britain although its population density is 10 percent higher. Comparing the history of the two sea-faring nations with respect to migration and colonization, it would seem likely that the Dutch population has included fewer lung cancer personalities likely to be fatally affected by socio-economic confinement. This conclusion is consistent with the findings of the Dutch historian Pieter Geyl (1965a, 1965b). He pointed out that the Dutch expansion was such a short-lived episode because "it was imposed on an inert or hostile majority by a tiny, but resolute minority" (Stone, 1965).

Finland has, next to Great Britain, the highest (76 percent of G.B.) lung cancer incidence of the world. This country may be described as having throughout centuries of domination by alien countries, maintained its language and culture, and finally achieved political independence from a vastly more powerful neighbor. Nevertheless its natives are hemmed in by a combination of unusual limitations due to circumstances of geography, language, economics and politics.

Japan has one of the lowest lung cancer rates in the world, 23 percent of that of Great Britain. Until 20 years ago it was a rigid, feudalistic society which hardly included a high contingent of independence-seeking individualists. This seems to explain why the high population pressure has not led to a corresponding incidence of lung cancer.

Iceland, the least urbanized and least industrialized of the countries listed, has also the lowest lung cancer rate.

West Berlin, it may be added, had in 1962, the highest incidence in the world, 111 per 100,000 of the male population. It is certainly most representative of a situation which tests the effect of drastic restriction of free movement on a naturally uninhibited and enterprising population (WHO, 1965).

There is another epidemiological fact which agrees with the psychobiological concept of lung cancer: *the far higher incidence of the disease in men than in women,* e.g., 58: 1 in the USA (1961); 7.4: 1 in Switzerland (1951-1960); 12:1 in Finland (1950) (U.S. Pub. Health Serv., 1964; Abelin, 1965). Two psychological facts contribute to this difference.

1. In all countries *men are subjected to greater stress than women*, if they are constitutionally endowed with a high need for individualistic independence. Most men work under conditions which they control only to a very limited extent, whereas married women have considerable independence in their homes. Working women, generally, do not expect the same level of achievement as men.

2. The latter point is related to a difference between male and female psychology which is pertinent for the lung-cancer-prone type of personality. As Erikson (1963) found, the different genital modalities of the sexes are manifest even in pre-adolescent children. When given material to construct on a table "an exciting movie scene" *boys* predominantly experienced the task as a challenge to overcome spatial limitations, e.g., they erected high buildings and set up traffic problems; *girls* predominantly accepted the given space on the table as the interior of a house, or they merely outlined the inner space by low walls. The accent was often on completely cheerful family scenes, or some intruder (man or animal) provided excitement, mostly humorous in character.

It seems obvious that the male mode involves a high sensitivity to restriction of freedom, whereas the female mode is apt to minimize the impact of such restrictions. Given the same constitutional need for individualistic freedom, men are therefore much more liable to feel frustrated to the extent of developing lung cancer.

3. Predisposition and Cigarettes in Lung Cancer

Several observers (Meerloo, 1944; McGovern, et al, 1959) have reported that the first physical symptoms of lung cancer are often preceded by *a severe, seemingly endogenous depression.* This prodromal period may last many months; in the case described above (Chapter V, B) at least 18 months. There is little likelihood that it will ever be possible to prove that the tumor becomes invasive at the time of the depression, but it is certain that the cancerous area may stay very small for a long time. This conscious depression at the beginning of lung cancer must be distinguished from the unconscious "somatized" depression which was described as an integral part of all cancer dynamics (Chapter V, B). Often the patients are aware of having suffered a serious loss before the malignancy developed in organs other than the lungs, but characteristically they continue to act "as if nothing had happened" until the physical symptoms of the tumor interfere, and even then they are apt to delay the seeking of medical help. (See Chapter III, Plate X, and Chapter V, B.) Severe physical handicaps are usually borne with stoic courage even by less outstanding cancer patients than those mentioned above, e.g., Freud, Taft, Wittgenstein and Batchelder.

The high psychological sensitivity to beginning lung cancer is understandable on the basis of the particular nature of the breathing function. It takes place at the borderline between conscious body control and unconscious physiological mechanisms; between the feeling of free will which man associates with his "voluntary" muscles, and the awareness of the limits set by the "autonomous" nervous system. It depends on circumstances which sphere leads at a given moment. The experience of encroachment on one's freedom is certainly expressed promptly by way of consciousness of breathing. In the case of lung cancer, the general human need for feeling in control of important situations has been a particular concern of the premorbid personality. The pathogenic situation, if not the tumor itself, is therefore apt to reach consciousness more easily than in the case of other body organs which are completely removed from willful action.[12]

Lung cancer represents a very striking contrast to bronchial asthma if one considers the two physical conditions as expressions of the underlying psychodynamics. The solid tumor takes the place of the lost adult object relationship (Chapter V, B), the asthmatic inflation with air marks the intense anxiety for the object which had initiated freedom from the maternal body.

Inasmuch as cancer reduces the area of contact with the "air of freedom" it resembles the effect of tuberculosis. There is, however, a profoundly significant difference. Tuberculosis tissue lives on oxidation like normal tissue; it is the regressive symbiotic process which threatens the life of the organism. Neoplastic tissue, however, derives its energy from the process of fermentation (Warburg, 1956) which preceded oxidation in evolution. Its independence from oxygen makes it a more autistic form of life. Thus, as the cancerous tissue expands in the lungs, it expresses on the microbiological as well as on the macroscopic level the existential situation of the patient: his frustrated striving for autistic freedom asserts itself symbolically at the expense of realistic survival.

The specific sensitivity of the lung-cancer-prone personality regarding encroachments on his free object control provides the explanation of the fact that he has been so often *dependent on cigarettes* before he became sick. As pointed out above cigarettes lend themselves to the need for substitute gratification in case of frustrated manipulative object relationships. Given *the high value of freedom in the "respiratory personality type"* the threshhold for experiences of frustration is apt to be low, and smoking cigarettes becomes particularly attractive.

For the lung cancer type, there is an important additional gratification provided by cigarettes. They lend themselves to *inhaling*. The latter practice has two significant components:
   a) the *act of inhaling as such* provides a feeling of liberation, even without the supporting effect of nicotine.
   b) the *sensation of the inhaled smoke, deep in the lungs* conveys an intensified feeling of control over a concrete object.

The conclusion appears reasonable that smoking and inhaling of cigarettes compensate for frustrations of the desire for free control of external objects. This is in keeping with the personality descriptions of cigarette smokers by other observers: Compared to non-smokers they change jobs more frequently, have a higher divorce rate, and have a poorer disciplinary record in the Armed Forces (U.S. Pub. Health Serv., 1964).

The role of cigarettes in Western materialistic culture is clarified further if one considers the breathing practices of the Yogi. For the latter, the control of breathing as such provides the experience of liberation from the bondage of the illusion of the separate ego, and of the reality of the material world in general. *All that the Yogi wants to relinquish, Western man wants to possess and control. He therefore endeavors to make the unsubstantial object of the lung more concrete by charging the inhaled air with smoke,* and paralyzing the cleansing mechanism of the bronchi. Nothing, perhaps, illustrates the magic illusions inherent in cigarette smoking more drastically than the fantastic prices which were paid for cigarettes after World War II in vanquished Germany.

The preceding interpretation of smoking and inhaling is consistent with the conclusions which Kissen (1964) drew from his clinical observations. He had observed previously that tuberculosis patients victimized by emotional deprivation recover better with the help of cigarette smoking (1960). In his studies of the personalities of lung cancer patients he was impressed by the fact that they have a poor outlet for emotional discharge, and that this difficulty is most pronounced among the non-inhalers. He therefore asked some pertinent questions: "Is it possible that non-inhalation represents a denial of outlet for emotional tension that inhalation is sometimes thought to provide? ...Does the giving up of smoking by persons who later become lung cancer patients also represent denial of an emotional outlet that had previously been utilized? ...Finally, if, as is suggested above, non-smoking in lung cancer patients represents denial of an emotional outlet that cigarette smoking provides, should it be expected that the poorer the outlet the less the cigarette consumption? Might it not be that the more effective the outlet the less the need for a tension reducer, and therefore the less the cigarette consumption? If, as is generally believed, cigarette smoking is used as a tension reducer is it not possible that it may be used by some with a poor emotional outlet *in an unconscious endeavor to find an outlet as well* as by some with a higher emotional outlet in a deliberate endeavor to ease tension (Kissen, 1964a, 1964b)? These formulations of Kissen point in the same direction as my own research. They are particularly noteworthy because his theoretical concepts of psychosomatic disease and his methods of research differ considerably from my own.

There are other observations which suggest that inhaling may serve as a specific prophylactic device through which the lung-cancer-prone personality defends himself against cancerogenic depression. Sir Ronald Fisher (1959), considered one of the world's greatest statisticians, analyzed the material on which Doll and Hill had based the conclusions that cigarettes cause cancer. When he separated inhalers from non-inhalers, he arrived at the uncontested result that *inhaling reduces the incidence of lung cancer by at least 10 percent.* He asked the unanswered question: "Should not these workers let the world know, not only that they discovered the cause of lung cancer (cigarettes), but also the means of its prevention (inhaling of cigarettes): How had the Medical Research Council the heart to withhold this information from the thousands who otherwise would die of lung cancer?"

Later investigators have not found the same phenomenon, perhaps because since the first Doll and Hill report in 1952, the cancer
scare has counteracted the tranquilizing effect of inhaling, but they
have confirmed that inhaling does not increase the risk for *heavy*
smokers (U.S. Pub. Health Serv., 1964). The latter are obviously most
dependent on the tranquilizing effects of cigarettes. It is therefore not
surprising that Hammond and Horn (1958) found in their follow-up
study of 187,783 men that among heavy cigarette smokers the lung
cancer incidence was *higher in the year after they stopped* than among
those who did not stop smoking: 198 to 157.1. Among those who
never were heavy smokers, and those who had stopped heavy smoking
more than 10 years, the rate was nearly the same: 60.5 to 57.6. The
authors found that those who had stopped heavy smoking recently had
done so because they felt sick. This, however, can also be interpreted as
meaning that they had smoked so heavily because they found their life
situation so hard to bear, and that they developed the cancer when even
heavy smoking did no longer help.[13]

The concept that cigarettes as tension reducers may have an anti-
cancerogenic effect is also supported by extensive experimental work
on cancer (Kavetsky, et al, 1966; Anderson, 1964).

It was found that the disturbance of cerebral control by experimental neuroses increases, and tranquilizing drugs decrease, the rate of
tumor growth. These observations are in keeping with many clinical
observations that cancers sometimes spread suddenly under the influence
of acute discouragement (Meerloo, 1954; Shapiro, 1963) and that the
patients hold their own under the influence of supportive physicians
(Mitchell, 1960; Beecher, 1962; Pendergrass, 1961; McKegney, et al,
1965).

The conclusion may be drawn that the rise of cigarette consumption in the 20th century represents a compensation for the frustrations
which are caused by the combination of infantile conditioning (Chapter
V, B) and of reduced freedom in adult life. Such unconscious wisdom
of the organism has been demonstrated experimentally in animals and
in human beings. Richter (1941) studied this phenomenon in rats. He
found that they are capable of choosing a diet so judiciously from 15
purified ingredients of food (fat, carbohydrate, protein, five minerals
and vitamins) that they ate between 15 and 40 percent less food per day
than those on a scientifically composed laboratory diet, but developed
equally well. He also found them capable of compensating for artificially inflicted diseases, e.g., diabetes, and pointed out similar accomplish-

ments in human patients. Davis (1928) had demonstrated even earlier that newly weaned infants are capable of choosing a healthy diet from a tray with different natural foods. The composition of the preferred diets varied greatly from one individual to another, including one infant afflicted with rickets who chose cod liver oil for the duration of the illness. Richter concluded from his observations: "Undoubtedly, most of the instances of peculiar appetites will be found to have dietary significance." Faulty dietary choices of human beings are often due to conditioning by parents, scientific theories and advertising. Applying this observation to the current campaign against cigarettes, it is certainly worth noting how many cigarette smokers have been clinging to their habit in the face of all the dire predictions that they risk lung cancer.

A constitutional basis of cigarette smoking was assumed by Seltzer (1963) on the basis of anthropometric data and by Eysenck (1965) on the strength of psychological research. He found that the "compulsive" cigarette smoker is an extrovert, that those who can stop are introverts without constitutional motivation. The latter, as demonstrated by the Rorschach tests, are also not cancer-prone. The same conclusion was reached, on the basis of a different method, by Coppen and Metcalfe (1964).

The preceding considerations suggest that *the frequent associa-tion between lung cancer and cigarette smoking may be analogous to the association between alcoholism and drinking.* A majority of people enjoy cigarettes and alcoholic beverages without ill effects, they enable them to cope more comfortably with the ordinary and special tensions of living. This effect is generally considered to be proven by the enor-mous sales of medically endorsed and prescribed tranquilizers. There is evidence that cigarette smokers have a slightly shorter life expectancy than non-smokers, *not only due to lung cancer but also due to other ordinary causes of death* (U.S. Pub. Health Serv., 1964). It remains to be seen, however, whether those who have taken tranquilizers for the same number of years will not also have a shorter life expectancy. One may surmise that those dependent on drugs may have been endowed with less vitality before they started to use them, and might have died even earlier without their chemical crutches.

Lung cancer patients and alcoholics are obviously not in the same constitutional group as the majority of those who use cigarettes and alcohol as tension releasers, their diseases are not the results of exces-sive use, but the excessive use is often the result of a specific disposi-tion and a specific environmental stress. True alcoholics are often, but not necessarily, heavy drinkers. Alcohol affects them differently from the average drinker. Instead of helping them to ease their tensions, it involves them in a vicious circle from which usually only the specialized help of Alcoholics Anonymous can extract them. *The lung cancer patient who has depended on cigarettes, becomes sick when they fail to compensate for his frustrations. Then he is reduced to self-expression through disease. It would be at this point that the histological changes found in the bronchi of smokers might become the starting area of malignant growth.*

The hypothesis is proposed that the personality type predisposed to develop lung cancer under specific stress is also most frequently predisposed to reach for cigarettes to reduce the stress which the modern world tends to cause for this personality type. Predisposition does not mean compulsion; there are for a certain percentage in this group powerful motivations to abstain: aesthetic, religious, moralistic, economic and, most recently, medical. This latter group seems to be very small, about 5 percent, in Anglo-Saxon countries. Abstainers comprise 40 percent of the male lung cancer mortality in Switzerland. This country is not noted for its polluted air, which has often been invoked as an explanation for lung cancer in non-smokers (Abelin, 1965).

The occurrence of lung cancer in non-smokers obviously does not exclude the possibility that cigarettes cause lung cancer among those who smoke. It appears very hazardous, however, to attempt the prevention of future lung cancer by abstaining from cigarettes. In view of the likelihood that cigarettes reduce the tensions of the lung-cancer-prone, the scare campaign in Anglo-Saxon countries is liable to have a pathogenic effect for those who feel robbed of an important experience of subjective freedom.

This point may be illustrated by a rather striking example (TIME, 1957). In 1933 Dr. Evarts Graham operated on a colleague diagnosed as having an abscess of the lung. He discovered, however, cancer and undertook the first total resection of a lung. This experience became the beginning of a successful career as a lung cancer surgeon. In 1951 he became suspicious of cigarettes as a cause of lung cancer. He retired from practice, stopped smoking, and devoted himself to experiments aimed at proving the causative role of cigarettes in animal experiments. Like everyone else, he failed to do so (U.S. Pub. Health Serv., 1964 — Report of the Surgeon General, p. 141). In 1957 he died of cancer of *both* lungs. His last visitor was the colleague on whom he had operated 24 years before. The latter had never stopped smoking, although his remaining lung was genetically as cancer prone as the one which had been resected. Furthermore, it had been subjected to 24 more years of cigarette smoking. Nevertheless, he survived another five years and did not die of cancer.

In the light of the psychodynamic theory of lung cancer the case appears to fit:

a) The *cancer* type is expressed in the individualistic devotion to the *control* of cancer, first through surgery, then through animal experimentation aiming at prevention.

b) The *lung* type is given to independent decision-making; e.g., first the undertaking of a new operation on the spur of the moment, then changing from surgery to laboratory work, and making himself independent from cigarettes on the strength of personal conviction before others had produced any of the material which has since been considered by many as compelling evidence against smoking.

c) *Frustration* brought on the lung cancer after he had failed to prove his hypothesis. He may also have been disturbed by the fact that his former patient had continued to smoke without a relapse.

The conclusion that cigarettes play only a contingent role in lung cancer, is in keeping with the observations of Passey (1962), one of the oldest researchers in the field of carcinogens. He found that the lung cancers of cigarette smokers, as well as those of nickel and chrome workers, developed after widely differing periods and intensities of exposure. The lack of a quantitative relationship between irritant and effect led Passey to the hypothesis that cigarette smoke and metal fumes act only as catalysts for an unknown carcinogenic agent. His conclusions have since been confirmed by Pike and Doll (1965), who found in Doll's own material that neither the amount smoked nor the age at starting affect the age of onset of the disease.

The material presented in this and the preceding chapter satisfies the postulates of the Surgeon General (U.S. Pub. Health Serv., 1964, p. 192) for an alternative to the cigarette theory of lung cancer. As formulated in his report there are three theoretical possibilities:

a) "there are genetic differences which make some individuals sensitive to a new environmental factor (not tobacco)"

b) "differences in constitutional make-up are not genetic but the result of differential exposure to some new factor that predisposes to lung cancer and creates the desire to smoke (cigarettes)"

c) "a mutation has produced an increased susceptibility and a desire to smoke."

"For the first two postulates a new environmental factor, other than tobacco, is required. Such a factor, it must be remembered, must be correlated with lung cancer as highly as are cigarettes, and also highly correlated with cigarette consumption. None has yet been found."

The first two postulates are satisfied by facts which previously have not been considered to be relevant. Most important is *the origin of the unexplained synchronous rise of excess cancer deaths and of cigarette consumption since 1900* (Fig. 3). It appears due to the fact that the population reaching cancer age at that time has been exposed increasingly to *the growing practice and success of artificial feeding* (bottle feeding and scheduling of breast feeding). As mentioned in the Surgeon General's report (p. 368 f), bottle feeding has been found related to cigarette smoking. Thus, differential exposure to artificial feeding would be the new environmental factor which predisposes to cancer in general, and creates the desire for cigarettes. Both phenomena are parallel manifestations of infantile conditioning, just as arteriosclerosis, neuritis and thirst are manifestations of diabetes mellitus, but not its cause.

The preceding step of separating general cancer liability from organ liability is in keeping with the findings of Tokuhata and Lilienfeld (1963) mentioned above. The genetic factor appears to be responsible for *organic and for functional manifestations in the respiratory organ, specifically for the tendency to smoke more cigarettes than those who are predisposed to become victims of other organ diseases.* A high correlation between constitutional disease predisposition and premorbid functional hyperactivity of the organ involved has impressed observers in the case of the locomotor system: arthritis and Parkinsonism (Booth, 1964a, 1946b, 1948). *Compulsive* smoking as a specific tendency in the lung disease group is suggested by its frequency in chronic bronchitis and emphysema since, in these conditions, the aggravation of the disease symptoms is an immediate experience of the patient (U.S. Pub. Health Serv., 1964). At least in the case of emphysema no causal relationship between cigarette smoking and the disease has been established (U.S. Pub. Health Serv., 1964).

In the case of lung cancer, smoking thus appears implicated as a secondary variable on two levels:

1. Cigarette smoking as such is highly correlated with general cancer disposition on account of infantile conditioning by artificial nursing methods.

2. Intensity of cigarette smoking is highly correlated with genetic disease liability of the lungs.

On both levels the habit appears to be a secondary variable. This interpretation of the facts is consistent with the great national differences in the frequency of lung cancer among non-smokers.

The rapid *increase of lung cancer since 1930* is another consequence of the genetic factor which predisposes to lung disease in general. As Berkson (1960) demonstrated, cancer is replacing tuberculosis as the cause of death in this genetic group. In spite of the spectacular rise of lung cancer the combined graphs of tuberculosis and lung cancer deaths add up to an actual slow, but steady decline since 1930. Others (Westergren, 1959; Barnes, 1960; Schwartz, 1960) have supported the evidence based on the mortality statistics with clinical observations proving that healed tubercular lesions are found frequently in cancerous lungs. It should be added that since 1930, pneumonia deaths also declined very impressively (Dubos, 1952) (Fig. 4). As a result the share of the lungs as the locale of fatal disease dropped from 28 percent in 1930 to 6.5 percent in 1962 (U.S. Vital Statistics). In other words, due to the improved control of infections, the population genetically predisposed for pulmonary disease has become subject to the increasing general cancer liability.

The preceding considerations provide the following concrete answers to the request of the Surgeon General for an alternative to the cigarette theory of lung cancer:

1. The *genetic* group sensitive to the new environmental factor is identical with the group which was formerly sensitive to the infectious agents of tuberculosis and pneumonia.
2. The *carcinogenic factor* is the result of two new conditioning processes to which the population has been subjected since the second half of the last century:
    a) the sharp reduction of biological interaction between organism and bacteria which was achieved by *modern hygiene.*
    b) the *change of object relations* by artificial infant feeding.
3. The change of object relations has found one expression in the growing popularity of *cigarettes* since bottle-feeding has become frequent and successful.
4. *Intensified cigarette smoking* is a functional characteristic of the genetic group predisposed to develop lung disease. It has a specific tranquilizing effect for this group.

5. *Lung cancer* develops as the result of frustration in a vital object relationship for which neither the psychobiological resources of the individual nor the tranquilizing effect of cigarettes can compensate. The connection between lung cancer and cigarettes is analogous to the connection between alcoholism and alcohol.

6. The *parallel between the rise of cigarette consumption and of cancer* has its origin in the conditioning of the population by bottle-feeding and modern hygiene. The result in adolescence is the desire for cigarettes; in later life, the cancer liability.

7. The *growing share of the lungs* in the rising cancer incidence is due to the fact that the population genetically predisposed to develop lung disease has been made cancer-prone by the measures which protect them against tuberculosis and pneumonia.

The preceding analysis of the epidemiological data accounts for the statistical association between cigarette smoking and lung cancer, it also disposes of the confounding aspects of the variables and contradicts the causal interpretation of the association.

4. *The Unconscious Motivation of the Cigarette Theory of Lung Cancer*

It seems a remarkable phenomenon that the nature of the link between lung cancer and cigarettes was not discovered earlier. There were many scientists who felt that the official American and British stance was based on inadequate scientific evidence. The Surgeon General's report admitted frankly that the statistical evidence did not jibe with a number of "confounding variables." The new interpretation is based on clinical facts which have been public knowledge for many years. The findings from the Rorschach study are not part of the new theory, they only encouraged the hypothesis that the understanding of cancer can be improved by the study of the personalities in whom the disease occurred.

The delay in recognizing the alternative to the causal cigarette theory of cancer suggests that rational evaluation was disturbed by an unconscious factor which had blinded prosecution and defense equally in the case of lungs against cigarettes. Berkson pointed out this complication in 1960: "... when the cause of a disease is not known, frequently it gets attributed to practices that are not approved, like the use of alcohol perhaps, or like smoking. Or it may be something else, ..." To give an example of my own: until the beginning of this century, masturbation was considered in many medical text books of the 19th century as a major cause of nervous and other illnesses until it was discovered that the practice is even more frequent than cigarette smoking today, and that *compulsive* masturbation is a *symptom* of the diseases of which it had been suspected to be the cause (Hare, 1962). It is hardly an accident that the two countries most strongly influenced by Puritanism have also produced the greatest public efforts to convict cigarettes of crime.

It is worth considering the reason behind the moral condemnation of cigarettes by Puritans. They emphasized work as the chief virtue. They were suspicious of *enjoyment of life* to such an extent that they even warned against this component of marital intercourse. They made people feel guilty about sexual desires and started the prosecution of masturbation. Smoking, like drinking, is not only unproductive, but even wasteful. Furthermore, both activities are reminders of the natural act of nursing, which is an enjoyable communication between infant and mother, not purely utilitarian. The latter emphasis was obviously the psychological preparation for the acceptance of bottle feeding in the industrial age. The emotional estrangement between parents and children which followed has rather increased the controversial role of cigarettes. Those who represent Puritanism in its modern form of scientific manipulation and utilitarian moralism insist that cigarettes have no legitimate place and are likely to be dangerous. Parents, therefore, insist that bottle feeding and hygienic raising of their infants fulfill all their duties. Children insisting on smoking proclaim implicitly that they have been deprived of the emotional satisfactions of the nursing period and refuse to allow themselves to be deprived also of the substitute joy of smoking. The majority of the population has now reached the stage where parents and children are at least united in asserting their rights for compensation for the deprivations imposed by a utilitarian civilization. *Cigarettes symbolize a defense of the basic symbiotic needs of man against the materialistic, individualistic values which dominate the public value system of modern culture.* This aspect of the problem explains the moralistic character of the current campaign against "the weed." Scientific critics of the verdict against cigarettes have been attacked with unprofessional hostility in respectable medical publications such as *The Lancet* (Berkson, 1962), not to mention the mass media. They are accused of being bought out by the industry, owning cigarette stocks, or trying to excuse their own lack of will power which makes them incapable of giving up their own "addiction."

There is a further cause for resentment against those who do not subscribe to the evilness of cigarettes. It deprives them of the pleasant fantasy that virtue has magic power. To stop the immoral practice would protect against lung cancer, the "just reward" of the "sinners." Perhaps it is this wishful thought that has made even the critics of the cigarette theory reluctant to press their point and to consider the full implications of the lung cancer epidemic.

The intensity of the "scientific" attack on cigarettes brings to mind the psychoanalytical observations on the "*screen memory*." The patient reports a traumatic incident, which is supposed to explain his condition, and insists that it is the ultimate cause of his illness. Actually, this maneuver protects the patient from facing some far more disturbing experience until he can take the latter in his stride. *The cigarette theory of lung cancer has fulfilled this protective function. As long as it promised to dispose of the threat of lung cancer, the far more alarming problem could be evaded which has expressed itself in the form of rising cancer deaths and of an 80-fold rise of cigarette consumption.*

There is no simple answer to the question of how the real causes of the cancer epidemic could be dealt with therapeutically. The contemporary population of industrial societies has been conditioned biologically and psychologically for the new way of life. It would have been impossible without two great triumphs of modern medicine: the control of microbial infections and success of artificial infant feeding. On the level of the individual, these developments created an analogous value system which aimed at control of the human and non-human environment, just as science aimed at "the conquest of nature." The transition from the symbiotic values of agricultural societies to the individualistic values of the present age appears to be an irreversible event in human evolution. It entailed cancer as its "social disease" just as the preceding age had been plagued predominantly by epidemic infections. Their conquest, it may be remembered, was not the result of scientific manipulation of the microbes alone, but also to a large extent the result of improved socio-economic conditions of the masses. What René Dubos wrote about tuberculosis may some day be written about cancer: "(The disease) is the consequence of gross defects in social organization, and of errors in individual behavior. Man can eradicate it without vaccines and without drugs by integrating biological wisdom into social technology and into management of everyday life." (1952) In a similar vein, Salk (TIME, 1965) recently predicted that his vaccine may be one of the last major successes of the laboratory in the medical field. He expects that the progress of the future will come from fuller understanding of social factors.

This long-range prospect for cancer therapy is difficult to accept by contemporary man who has been led to believe in the unlimited possibilities of scientific manipulation of nature. The romanticized stories of microbe hunters, magic bullets and miracle drugs have led to the expectation of a dramatic "break-through" in the "war against cancer." The truth is likely to be different. To get rid of the problem we will have to work patiently at the complex job of social and cultural change. Against this painful insight, the cigarette controversy provided a protective smoke screen. As so often happens, the screen memory correctly marked the area of the problem: the nursing period of personality development. It concealed, however, the fact that prophylaxis would have to start at birth, properly speaking in the nursing period of the child's parents.

Summary

The *predisposition* to develop lung cancer is created by genetic and infantile conditioning. Localization in the lungs is characteristic of individuals endowed with specific striving for independence from their given environment. The neoplastic character of the disease process is the liability of the so-called anal character which frequently results from the unnatural methods of modern infant care.

The *disease* develops at the point when the predisposed individual experiences the irretrievable loss of hope for attaining the level of independence for which he has been striving according to his personality make up.

The *rapid increase* of lung cancer in modern industrialized populations is explained by the fact that cancer has been replacing tuberculosis as a general disease disposition. This change is consistent with the cultural conditioning of the population. The socio-economic progress did not eliminate the frustrations of independent strivings to which the individual of the "respiratory type" is most sensitive. *Cigarettes function as tension releasers for him*, the more frustrated he feels, the greater is his tendency to smoke and to inhale. There is some evidence that smoking has prophylactic value. Cigarette smoke does not act as a physical carcinogen inasmuch as neither time nor quantity of exposure is related to the onset of the disease. *After* a frustrating life situation has brought about the carcinogenic depression (Chapter V) the smoke may operate as a catalyst for the neoplastic process.

The causal interpretation of the association between cigarettes and lung cancer is explained as a psychological phenomenon. The concentration on a physicalistic theory of lung cancer provides an unconscious screen against awareness of the disturbing psychosocial roots of the rising frequency of cancer in other organs and among children under smoking age.

IX

The Psychological Problems of
Cancer Therapy

A. The New Concept of Cancer

Traditionally, cancer therapy has been guided by the image of a human body serving as an unwilling host to a stealthy and murderous invader. Anybody seemed liable to become a victim of a sneak attack. This concept has led to a war-like approach to the problem of malignancies. "Destroying the invader" is the common aim of most research and of the various surgical, radiological and chemical devices of therapy. At the same time, the stealth of cancer development has given rise to a widespread paranoia which tries to mobilize public opinion against such popular purveyors of pleasure as sex and cigarettes, on the basis of circumstantial evidence. The lowering of scientific standards corresponds to that of judicial standards in times of war. Also, in analogy with war psychology, the experience that the enemy has been gaining steadily over the last hundred years has led to increasingly radical methods of destructiveness and propaganda.[14] The persistent lack of success of this approach has led a minority in the medical profession to counsels of moderation, e.g., George Crile, Jr. (1955), but in a desperate war the moderates have little chance to gain an effective majority.

The re-evaluation of the known clinical facts in the light of psychodynamic research has led to a very different image of the cancer patient. Far from being the victim of a foreign invader, he reveals himself as a clear example for John Donne's statement that each man is "his own executioner." The unconscious self-destruction through the tumor is the ultimate form of the dominant striving for *control* over the object which he has valued most highly, in contrast to the symbiotic mutuality of the object relationships of tuberculosis patients (Chapter III). The ultimate defeat of the extraverted striving for control of the external object leads to the creation of its symbolic substitute inside of the frustrated organ (Chapter V). The ruthless growth of the latter, unless stopped by therapy, represents the final triumph of the narcissistic function over the less-valued potentialities of the organism (Chapter VIII).

The conflict between the healthy and the sick functions can certainly be described as a war, but it is a civil war rather like the kind which sometimes follows the return of a vanquished army to native soil. Having failed to gain control over foreign territory, the defeated forces try to dominate in their own country. Recognition that the invasive growth represents the desperate self-expression of the patient calls for a new rationale of therapy. It may save the organism, or the nation, to destroy an alien invader; but if the disturbance is caused by excesses of a vital part of the biological or political body, re-integration and not radical destruction is called for.

The consequences of this insight for therapy are simple in theory. The proliferation of neoplastic cells results from the disturbed communication between the diseased organ and its former objects (Chapter VIII, A). The patient, therefore, needs to be given back satisfactory objects, or he may reorganize his object relationship so that the diseased function reduces its demands. The physician does not have much control over the object world of the cancer patient, and the cancer patient is not easily influenced, even in his younger years. To some extent this is true for all somatic diseases; in the case of cancer, it is intensified.

There is, furthermore, an additional obstacle to rational therapy specific to cancer. The patients and most modern doctors are committed to the value system of industrial culture. Constitutional disposition on the one hand, academic indoctrination on the other hand, both create a bias for problem-solving by way of unilateral control over the object of their endeavors. This leads to an unconscious clash of interests where the object is a malignant growth. The physician tries to comply with the overt request, but he is up against the unconscious motivation of the patient for whom the tumor symbolizes the part of reality which he had been most eager to control previous to his illness. This conflict creates an unfavorable setting for therapy and its consequences are well known.

First of all, cancer patients are particularly *reluctant to seek medical help*. Goldsen, Gerhard and Handy (1957) investigated the reasons for the delay and discovered the following paradoxical facts:

1. Patients seek diagnosis more promptly for seemingly harmless symptoms than for those which are apparent to others.
2. Chronic cancer worriers who know a lot about cancer are most inclined to delay in seeking help.

These points have been confirmed in a study which Gold (1964) made of 100 women with breast cancer and 50 with benign lesions of the breast. He found that at the time of the first examination the median diameter of the lump was 6 cm in the cancerous, and 2.5 cm in the non-cancerous group.

The other consequence of cancer psychology for inadequate therapy is the *secretiveness* of the patients regarding the circumstances associated with the onset of the illness. The motivation has been explained as the result of guilt feelings engendered by the evidence that the striving for anal control has failed—the final defeat of an endeavor which dominated the life of the patient.

Autistic personality, belated asking for help, secretiveness and guilt feelings all contribute to the lack of understanding cancer patients feel they get from their doctors. Before science had become so confident that it gave medicine the power to conquer natural phenomena, physicians had seen their task as supporting the healing powers of the sick organism. Faith in the "vis medicatrix naturae" made them observant of all the symptoms which suggested opportunities for cooperation. The causative role of losses and the state of depression used to be common knowledge (Kowal, 1953; Kavetsky, et al, 1966; LeShan, 1959) instead of being either ignored or considered secondary to the physical process. Also, the observations of the disappearance of cancer after a severe infection were not dismissed as cases of mistaken diagnoses. In the 20th century, Coley (Nauts, Fowler, Bogatko, 1953; J.A.M.A., 1934) stood alone with his life work devoted to utilize streptococcus vaccines in order to change the cancerous reactivity of the organism. It is a telling example for the "physicalist" bias of modern medicine that there has been practically no follow-up of this truly biological approach, although Coley obtained complete remission in 270 inoperable cases. This figure is particularly significant because as head of the Bone Tumor Service of the New York Memorial Hospital he saw predominantly sarcomas which are less responsive to his toxin therapy than soft tissue tumors. In the light of the new evidence for the pervasive difference between the pregenital dynamics of cancer, and the genital dynamics of infectious disease, the observations of the old physicians and the therapeutic successes of Coley appear plausible. In certain patients, apparently, a change in the balance of power between the instinctual reactions can be achieved by means of a powerful infectious stimulus. Tinbergen's (1955) book on instincts is full of examples for the fact that the result of exposure to competing "instinct releasers" depends not only on the internal condition (sex hormones and hunger, for example) of the organism, but also on the relative intensity of the corresponding environmental signals.[15]

The concentration of modern scientists on external methods of destroying the tumor is only partly explained by the physicalistic rationale of the age. It appears motivated also by the psychological reaction to the personality of the cancer patient. The physician is called upon to treat a disease which so far has made consistent gains against the tremendous mobilization of intellect, money and public opinion undertaken to cure it. He is therefore uncertain of his chances for success even under the ideal circumstances of early discovery, and in all too many cases he finds himself under the additional handicap of being called belatedly, or even too late, to do anything. In view of what psychiatry has learned about unconscious perception it seems likely that many surgeons and radiologists are, at least unconsciously, aware of the autistic resistance of their patients, particularly in proportion to their own pregenital orientation. Gold, in the article mentioned above, found that 17 percent of the physicians who had examined his patients before him, had failed to recognize the malignancy. This figure coincides with the cancer-prone percentage of the American population.

Anxiety about therapeutic success on the side of the medical profession enhances necessarily the modern tendency to meet power with power. The result is the growing radicalism of therapeutic methods which caused Sutherland (1957a), the psychiatrist of Memorial Hospital in New York, to raise the question whether cancer therapy should be made "less extensive and less radical." He had realized that the men of medicine had at this time become more successful in saving lives than in assisting their patients in making the lives saved also worth living. In many cases the delay in seeking help is certainly motivated by fear of disfigurement and disabilities. Thus a vicious circle of medical aggressiveness and cancerous resistance is set in motion. It seems to be an unnecessary complication of cancer therapy. Experienced cancer surgeons, e.g., George Crile, Jr. in his book *Cancer and Common Sense,* have tried to set public opinion straight regarding the increasingly terrifying popular image of cancer (Stehlin and Beach, 1966).

The new concept of cancer indicates that this disease cannot "strike anyone at any time." It is the specific liability of persons in whom autistic (anal) needs predominate over symbiotic (genital) needs. This type of person becomes depressed after defeat in conflict with corresponding pressures of the social environment. The depression becomes somatized in the form of cancer and entails specific guilt feelings. Rational therapy requires that not only the physical symptom be treated, but that the patient be helped in finding a constructive solution for the conflict which caused the depression. Support in meeting the social problem involves, in addition to the practical issue, therapeutic encouragement for the neglected symbiotic potentiality of the patient. That this change in the balance of instincts may be obtained in some cases even by purely biological methods has been suggested by the successes of Coley's vaccine. The main point of the new concept of cancer therapy is the recognition of the role which the personality of the patient plays in producing as well as overcoming a malignant reaction.

B. *The Destruction of the Tumor*

Recognition of the tumor as the physical symptom of a depression implies that it is the unconscious equivalent of a conscious suicidal act. Removal of the tumor is therefore essentially an emergency measure analogous to the medical or surgical steps undertaken in cases of incomplete suicidal attempts. Physical action in order to remove the self-created instrument of self-destruction is a vital necessity, but as in all other forms of suicide attempts, the future of the patient depends on the subsequent development of his life situation. If the latter does not change for the better, the attempt will be repeated consciously or unconsciously.

The observations of Stengel (1962) on suicide as a *social signal* are equally pertinent for cancer. Family and friends are made aware that the patient is in serious distress. Even though they may be unaware of the causes, their efforts to be helpful often seem to boost the morale of the patient, to inspire him with new courage and hope. Thus he may take a new lease on life to good advantage and not become a repeater. Unfortunately in a number of cases the despair of the patients is well founded. Nobody is interested in giving them a second chance. Cancer is so frequent that probably most readers will be able to think of pertinent examples from personal experience. A particularly crass illustration may be taken from Beecher (1962). A woman was told by a relative "the truth" immediately after having undergone surgery, namely that the tumor was inoperable. Within the hour, the patient went into shock and died a few hours later. One may assume that the hasty communication had not been motivated by good will since the physical condition of the patient would have allowed at least a few more months of life.

Fortunately, family and friends are not the only resources of emotional support for the operated cancer patient. The physician can be particularly helpful because he is not likely to be personally a part of the psychological situation which brought about the cancerogenic depression. All depressions involve guilt feelings for the patient and those close to him and a vicious circle is apt to develop. The therapeutic advantage of the physician, however, is frequently not used because modern medical training has become concerned nearly exclusively with the prolongation of physical life even when the time gained is psychologically meaningless. In the field of neoplastic disease the triumphs of surgical techniques have made this problem most clear, particularly when life can be made bearable only by lobotomy or its more refined versions. As Harry Stack Sullivan remarked about the original use of psychosurgery in psychiatry, it was not therapy but "fractional euthanasia." Even aside from psychosurgery, due to the conditions of his work, the surgeon is very limited regarding possibilities of establishing a helpful psychological relationship with his patients. Nevertheless, it was a surgeon, D. Lang Stevenson (1964), to whom we owe a most illuminating essay on the interplay of biology and psychology in cancer.

Radiologists are generally in a much more favorable situation to become familiar enough with the personalities of their patients to appreciate and consider their psychological needs. The contact is prolonged and the physical techniques less dramatic and absorbing than in surgery. Thus, on the basis of large clinical experiences, Mitchell (1960) and Smithers (1964) in England, and Pendergrass (1961) in America, arrived independently at conclusions which bear out those which the pioneers of psychological cancer studies had drawn from psychiatric explorations (Evans, 1926; Meerloo, 1954) and from psychological tests (Tarlau and Smalheiser, 1951; Gengerelli and Kirkner, 1954; LeShan and Worthington, 1956). I quoted Smithers earlier (Intro. p. 3). Pendergrass wrote that the physician "must be aware that many of the signs and symptoms manifested by the sick person are attempts at adaptation and expression rather than the disease itself. Such thoughts must be clearly kept in mind, otherwise the attempts at therapy will deprive the patient of defenses without making more suitable ones available at the same time. This commonly happens in present day medicine, when the specialist directs attention to one group of symptoms and ignores their significance for the total adjustment of the patient. Over the years, many have been unable to evaluate the constitutional factors observed by good clinicians. One wonders whether the glamor of the scientist and the dissection of the cell and its components has not led us into a path away from important environmental influences.... There are many ways of treating cancer, but one thing is certain; if the program of therapy includes a high level of cooperation and consultation at all levels, the patient will get a better deal."

C. *"The Truth"*

The preceding resumé of the conclusions of Pendergrass explains the author's position regarding the much discussed problem of whether the patient should be told the truth about his physical condition. Pendergrass is justified in doing so because in contrast to the relative mentioned above, he is able to tell the *whole* truth. The physical measures are not tickets in a lottery which give the sick a series of statistical chances for being found operable, for surviving five years and for dying eventually of a non-cancerous cause. The whole truth includes the assurance that the patient is an integral agent in the process of recovery, and that the physician is his ally in developing and maintaining his morale. This attitude of the physician also sets an example specifically for the autonomy-minded cancer patient. He does not act as if his profession had put him into a position of unilateral power and as consequence does not provoke the dangerous defensiveness of cancer patients against outside interference. More than in psychotherapy, healing of cancer is achieved by the shared efforts of the therapist and the patient.

The question of whether cancer patients *want* to know the truth has been answered so differently by equally experienced physicians that the logical conclusion seems obvious: *it depends on the personality of the physician.* Jaffe and Slote (1958) demonstrated in a clinical experiment that the same patients acknowledge or deny their illness according to their perceptions of the attitudes of the interviewers. There are good reasons for the assumption that unconsciously the patients know their conditions always, and most of them consciously, too. For many, however, the disease and the situation behind it represent enough of an inner strain that they avoid discussion with outsiders who add to it, such as visitors who cannot face cancer due to a personal phobia, and physicians who are embarrassed by the uncertainty of professional success. Even cancer patients who know that they are incurable take their condition well in the large majority of cases (Crile, 1955). Some deny knowledge of their condition for reasons which have nothing to do with their feelings about themselves. Sutherland (1957b), for instance, reported the following incident of a very rich man who was approaching death in a cancer hospital. He had not made a will and because of this the family wanted the doctor to tell the patient the truth. The man, however, accused the doctor of lying and insisted he was suffering from infectious hepatitis, that he was not in danger of dying. It seems most likely that the patient was well aware of the insincere motivation for being told the self-evident truth. So he told the doctor quite correctly as far as the true issue was concerned, "You are lying. You don't want to tell me about my condition which is obvious, but you want to make me talk to my lawyer, and that is none of your business."

Beyond the interpersonal variables of honesty in communications with patients, there is one important point about "the truth" which should not be forgotten, and that is the unpredictable course of the disease. There can be no question that a pessimistic prognosis can have a catastrophic effect on these patients (Meerloo, 1954). Cancer entails guilt feelings and depression due to its own dynamics. In a denial of hope the sick experience rejection, an eagerness of the environment to get rid of a frustrating and often guilt-provoking "case." Thus, the pathogenetic effect of the original object loss is increased, whereas some form of psychological encouragement changes the inner balance of healthy and malignant tendencies for the better.

A telling example was that of the composer, Bela Bartok. He had a highly respected position in Hungary but left for reasons of political idealism. He found little appreciation in America. He developed leukemia and was close to death in a hospital when he received a very important commission to compose a concert. He recovered and fulfilled the contract before he suffered a final relapse (Heinsheimer, 1952).

Shapiro (1963) reported on a man who had orange-sized masses of sarcoma in the neck, axilla, groin, chest and abdomen, requiring draining of the pleura every second day. After one day of Krebiozen medication the tumor masses shrank to half the original size. He could be discharged and held his own until he had a relapse two months later upon reading negative reports on Krebiozen in the newspapers. The physician reassured him and gave him injections of saline solution described as double strength of Krebiozen. Again he became ambulatory and symptom free for over two months. Then he read that the American Medical Association had taken a stand against Krebiozen. Within a few days the patient relapsed and returned to the hospital where he died within less than 48 hours.

There are cancer patients with such inner strength that they can take a very pessimistic prognosis in their stride. For instance, Brian Hession, an Anglican clergyman, was operated for lung cancer at the age of 45. He was given three days to live, but he recovered and started an organization, Cancer Anonymous. In its service he lived through seven more years and four more operations before he finally died. He was convinced that faith and determination can help cancer patients to become cured or at least to endure their disease.

The topic of so-called "spontaneous regressions" is much neglected in modern research. Although there are about 176 well-observed cases in the literature according to Everson and Cole (1966), who estimate that they occur once in 80,000 to 100,000 cases, many physicians hold on to the "scientifically untenable...current belief that all cancers are irreversible, that all observations of spontaneous regressions are to be dismissed as mistaken diagnoses (Smithers, 1964)." The power of this kind of thinking is so strong in the case of cancer that it may be safely assumed that many are not written up for publication because physicians and journals are notoriously reluctant to become publicly associated with "far-out views." I have been told of these cases by surgeons I trust, and there are others who have had enormous experience who assert truthfully that they never observed a spontaneous remission. Considering what has been found about the influence of the physician on his patients it seems very believable that the dogmatic surgeon is least likely to get his patient over the shock that the tumor proved inoperable.

The doctrine of the irreversible character of cancer and its purely physical causes is in keeping with the modern physicalistic concept of science. "Spontaneous regression" means recovery without demonstrable (meaning "physical") cause, a heretical notion in the case of a "physical" disease like cancer. Heresies sometimes prove to be anticipations of orthodoxies of the future. The psychiatrist reading the current literature on cancer is reminded vividly of the literature on "dementia praecox" in the twenties. Then and now the majority opinion was that the disease runs an irreversible course to mental death in an institution. Then and now scientific research was directed toward the discovery of some biochemical fault inside the organism which caused cellular deterioration, assumed in "dementia praecox" and visible in cancer. Then and now there were publications about "spontaneous remission." Others indicated that psychodynamic processes were involved in the disease which, if understood and used intelligently, could influence the allegedly irreversible process therapeutically. Then and now the majority opinion decided that the successes only proved that the diagnoses had been wrong. Today "dementia praecox" is as antiquated a diagnosis as demon possession and has been replaced with the psychodynamic concept of schizophrenia. It is still a serious disease but irreversible only to the extent to which the pathogenetic conditions and the attitudes of the physicians prove to be so. Many schizophrenics today make better "reality adjustments" than so-called "normal" people, not only with the help of the new physical therapies, but also because physicians have learned to give their patients a second chance after a "break down."

The many parallels between the development of the "dementia praecox" concept, and the present struggle for a psychodynamic cancer theory are manifestations of the same basic fact of cultural evolution. The majority of physicians and scientists is deeply indoctrinated by the cultural value system of its period in history. The Kraepelinian school of psychiatry defended the Victorian concept of life; then the impact of the socio-economic revolution of World War I with its consequences ended both. In the aftermath, there came recognition that schizophrenic symptoms result from the interaction between persons born with a specific vulnerability and corresponding psychological demands on their human environment. The contemporary physicalistic view of cancer defends the materialistic concept of life which has led the industrial societies to the completely dehumanized possibility of atomic war. The psychodynamic study of cancer is part of the re-awakened search for a new humanism among many individuals and groups. The whole truth about cancer transcends, in any patient, his personal problems and involves all who participate in making the present world. "Send not to ask for whom the bell tolls; it tolls for thee."

D. Therapy

The discovery of having cancer has, for the patient, the same effect as having attempted suicide. It is well known that in many cases such attempts are not repeated even though the circumstances motivating the act do not change (Stengel, 1962). It seems that the realistic confrontation with the existential issue is apt to bring about a conscious or unconscious change of the inner attitude. Having acted out to a certain extent his self-destructive tendencies the would-be suicide becomes willing to sacrifice part of his original autistic demands. In the case of cancer the salutary reorientation may be aided by the operation itself since it removes part of or the whole organ which represented the over-valued function in the autistic relationship with the world. This effect must not be understood as the result of the physical reduction of the organ. Except in the case of endocrine glands, physiological consequences are not conceivable. The psychological effect of a symbolic sacrifice, however, seems plausible since the cancerous organ had played an important part in the premorbid life of the patient. This aspect of cancer surgery is suggested particularly by those cases of "spontaneous remission" which sometimes follow an exploratory operation revealing an inoperable tumor. Cancer is, after all, a specific form of depression and it is known that surgical intervention produces remissions occasionally in cases of purely psychotic depression (Titchener and Levine, 1960).[16]

The potential effect of an inner change on the prognosis of the disease may suggest to some psychotherapeutic enthusiasts that "deep psychotherapy" should be instituted in all cases as a prophylactic post-operative measure. Such a conclusion would be highly unrealistic. Somatization of a conflict expresses dynamics which are ingrained in the physical structure of the organism, in that layer of the unconscious which was never conscious, to quote Sherrington's *Man on His Nature* (1941). Although it is evident that under the impact of a realistic existential encounter the power balance in the personality structure can be influenced, it would be an impossible undertaking to try to imitate such encounters across a desk or the head-end of a couch. Even in the case of functional neuroses and psychoses, so much closer to the past and present consciousness of the patient, the results of deep psychotherapy are limited by the uncontrollable contingencies of the patient's inner resources and external situation as well as the personality of the therapist.

The observations of Meerloo (1954) indicate that there is a possibility of systematic therapy on a psychoanalytical basis in cancer, but we do not know enough about the total situation involved to estimate what special conditions supported the work of an unusually gifted and experienced therapist. He, himself, felt that his results could not be generalized. The same should be said about the incidents of religious cancer healings reported from Lourdes and America (Braden, 1954). It may very well be that the powerful impact of collective emotions on a particularly receptive person may, in rare cases, have the effect of changing even biological reactions, comparable to the *modus operandi* of infections and of Coley's vaccine.

From the borderland between functional and organic processes an additional method of changing the response of the patient should be mentioned. In 1962 Koroljow published two cases in which he had treated depressions caused by inoperable malignancies (cervix and metastatic melanoma) with insulin coma. In both cases not only the depressions, but also the malignancies disappeared. The author, incidentally, did not consider the psychological aspects of cancer, but only the possibility that the insulin coma had influenced the metabolism of the cancer cells by increasing the oxygen concentration in the surrounding media.

Having acknowledged the possible, but uncontrollable influence of inner change on cancer, it must be stressed that it would be utter folly to *expect* such change from these constitutionally autistic and usually older patients. The primary responsibility of the therapist is to accept them as they happen to be, and try to help them within the given limitations of personality and reality situations. Observations such as those of McKegney (1965) demonstrate that opportunity for positive object relationships prolongs life, and their frustration by materialistic management ends it abruptly. One of his patients suffering from Hodgkin's disease, had found a new purpose in life in the hospital. Inspired by her experience, she gave speeches to groups of medical students, chaplains and social workers and communicated to them the realistic needs of those she termed "so-called incurables." She was improving physically when it was decided to transfer her to a convalescent home prior to her own home, a dismal prospect because her disease had been preceded by divorce. Faced with the loss of her newly found vocation she died the morning of the transfer of a massive, endogeneously caused hematemesis.

E. Social Therapy

The first psychological study of cancer by Evans already expressed the opinion that the ultimate result of operations seemed to depend on the successful substitution of a new object for the lost one. Ideally it is the medical therapist who should support the patient in his efforts to become once more a participant in the world from which he had withdrawn in despair. This support begins with the post-operative care provided by the medical staff, nurses and visitors. The emotional needs of the patient must be considered, not only the proper working of the technical equipment supporting the vital organs. Unfortunately, the high development of the technical side of surgery makes so many demands on the attention of the hospital personnel that there is little opportunity for the human aspect of the contacts between the patient and the many people who are busy around him. This situation does not pertain uniquely to the cancer patient, but it is particularly bad for him because in addition to the physical pain and anxiety he is depressed.

In 1961 the Trustees of the American Medical Association decided that the emotional deprivation of the modern hospital patients called for remedial action. Since the clergy is the only group specifically experienced in helping distressed human beings, their cooperation was solicited. A nation-wide program of regional conferences between physicians and clergy was organized and met with enthusiastic response from both groups. It holds a fair promise of being put into practice and giving cancer patients a better chance for psychological and social rehabilitation, at least those who belong to some religious group. Others will have to rely on the affection of family and friends; this should become more possible in proportion to the spreading of psychological knowledge about cancer patients.

All too often cancer patients are isolated from full human communication not only by the technological apparatus and mentality of modern medical care, but also by the embarrassment of the psychological situation. For the reasons discussed previously, cancer is surrounded, for too many people, with the same aura of evil formerly associated with venereal diseases. With the change of the cultural values from genital to anal emphasis, cancer has become the new "social disease," essentially for the same reasons. Each case of venereal disease originated somewhere in a person who failed to integrate his or her sexuality fully with the worship of fertility; each case of cancer proves that the person failed to integrate his or her anal instincts with the worship of the autonomy and freedom of the individual. Unconsciously, the cancer patient is experienced not only as the victim of a disease, but as a person who has betrayed the cause of the materialistic ideals of modern man.

It is a somewhat ironical, but psychologically meaningful, fact that materialistic scientific medicine should turn at this point officially to the ministers of religion for help. As we saw previously, organized religion originally developed from the need to organize society around the biological laws which govern fertility and made individual comfort and security matters of secondary importance. Materialistic ethics of industrial society developed from the preoccupation with the needs of the individual, first for personal salvation of the soul and then for the personal comfort and freedom of secular existence. Cancer then developed as the specific risk incidental to the pursuit of the new values.

The human needs of cancer patients *can* be met by the clergy. It is fitting that these needs were understood and made part of a practical program by a minister whose own existence was deeply involved in his tragic love for a woman who died of cancer (Boisen, 1960). Consciously, Anton Boisen had developed the widely accepted program for clinical training of the clergy as the result of his own experience as an inmate of a mental hospital.

He had been supported in his research on the significance of that episode by his devotion to Alice Batchelder who had been unable to be more to him than a loyal friend and whose death from breast cancer had coincided with the completion of his book.

Boisen taught that the sick need "to be restored to the human fellowship" and this purpose is best accomplished by encouraging them to *communicate their life histories.* This calls for empathetic human interest in the patient, and, obviously, for time, although not as much as the reader might think. Given the proper attitude of the minister, his visits should result in a chronological sequence of "personal" and "medical" events which makes their interrelationship obvious without probing into the unconscious dynamics. The latter, if used by the unwise and inexperienced, whether professional or amateur, often distracts attention from the problems about which something can be done. In view of the recent appeal for help from the clergy, it is most unfortunate that the glamor of scientific manipulation has influenced the current methods of pastoral clinical training far too greatly. The participants in these courses tend to become preoccupied with the search for psychoanalytical motivations in themselves and in their patients. All this leads to disregard for overt biographical communication and thus to disregard for the dignity of the person.

Excessive concern with psychoanalytic interpretation has not only interfered with the implementation of Boisen's insight into the clinical training of the clergy; medical training has been equally affected. Adolf Meyer, in the first part of the present century, taught the importance of psychobiological observation to thousands of students and attendants of psychiatric meetings in America. He emphasized the value of synchronizing the two sequences of biographical and medical events as a rational approach to the understanding of the interrelationship between the different spheres of life, but in reading recent case histories one finds little evidence of Meyer's influence. Often the data are all there, but the author made no connections.

The separation of body and soul is so deeply ingrained in the Western mind that not only physicians, but also the patients themselves are surprised when they are given a demonstration of synchronicity between life experience and disease. Most people tend to repress all reminders that the psyche is involved in far more of life than conscious thinking and those spheres of self-expression which are close to conscious experience and control such as the oral, anal and sexual functions. The persistent dichotomy of medical thinking after more than 60 years of psychoanalysis seems incomprehensible, but then it must be remembered that Freud himself had seen in his discoveries mainly the opportunity to expand the power of the conscious ego into that sphere of the psyche which contained the experiences which had been originally conscious and then become repressed. For him there remained always the rock-bottom of the organic sphere devoid of psychological meaning. He certainly expressed the hope that science would eventually learn to modify this stumbling-block, but that it would have to be the other science which analyzes and manipulates "matter." The history of Freud's own cancer shows the psychoanalytical scotoma for psychobiological synchronicity. Although it is documented in the three-volume biography by Ernest Jones, nobody seems to have attributed any significance to the sequence of his daughter Sophie's death, the development of the "death instinct" as a metaphysical concept, followed by the death of his grandson and his depressive reaction to it and his own cancer. Considering this lack of perceptiveness in Freud and his disciples, it is important to keep in mind that selectivity and distortion of memory are no less a liability of less sophisticated cancer patients and observers. Dates must be carefully checked even when they concern rather recent events.

Restoring patients to the human fellowship through listening to their life histories does not require any psychiatric training, and only a certain awareness of the generic idiosyncrasies of the cancer group. Their need for individualistic self-sufficiency involves communication problems, particularly their tendency to be secretive about certain aspects of their lives. It should be remembered, however, that this secretiveness serves in most cases only the purpose of protecting themselves against attempts to interfere in their private worlds. Their illness itself is the result of fate having defeated them, so they are wounded and defensive against judgmental attitudes and also against meddling attempts to be helpful in word or deed without being asked. The modern enthusiasm about "doing something about it" makes members of the helping professions oblivious to the healing powers of straight fellowship. The autism of cancer patients does not mean that others do not matter, only that the capacity to communicate with others is more limited than those of the symbiotic, genital type. For this very reason, the possible relationships are also more vitally important to them than for the type who can find substitutes more easily.

It might be suspected that ministers would be particularly tempted to be carried away by missionary zeal, either in the direction of helping in a secular way or through spiritual conversion. For them, as well as for psychotherapists, it is difficult to recognize that certain psychological attitudes are so deeply conditioned by heredity and infantile conditioning that they must be accepted; although the patients may even be capable of seeing intellectually that a change would be desirable. Most members of the clergy, however, seem to be levelheaded as a result of their extensive professional experience with human limitations. I have spoken three times to large interdenominational groups about cancer psychology and was very favorably impressed by the high level and pertinence of the long discussions which followed.

It should be made explicit that all these considerations apply to all cancer patients, those with a favorable prognosis and those considered terminal cases. Perhaps the latter are even more entitled to the reconciliation with the world which has dealt them, often unwittingly, a deadly blow. LeShan (1961) has given much attention to psychotherapy with those who experience particular difficulty in facing death, a remarkably small group in a hospital for incurable cancer patients. He found that even those handicapped by more than average psychological difficulties could be helped to make the ends of their lives meaningful for themselves and their families. To those who criticized this work as a waste of time he replied that "the search for the self—in another age one might have called it the growth of the soul—is not relevant to the fluttering of leaves on a calendar."

There is another form of professional psychotherapy which in some cases removes the pain which some terminal patients undergo. This is hypnosis as developed by Sacerdote (1964). It is included under "Social Therapy" because its effectiveness is based on the establishment of human rapport even though the method operates through unconscious interpersonal channels. This process presupposes the need of the patients to be met psychologically. It seems important to stress the power of this need because they are easily forgotten in the preoccupation with the *physical* condition and the *physical* pain. Pure physical therapy is tempting because it avoids the greater demand on time and mind which go with human concern. To give in to this temptation, however, means a betrayal of human responsibility for our neighbor. Fractional euthanasia through brain surgery or narcotics may dull the pain of the patient and the conscience of the physician, but it is not the best medicine can do for the human problem of cancer.

Treatment of cancer patients must be based upon the recognition that the tumor represents an unconscious suicidal attempt. Removal of the tumor may have an incidental healing effect on the underlying depression, but this result should not be relied upon. Each patient, regardless of the nature of the tumor classification and surgical findings, should be treated as a person who needs attention to his implicit need for re-establishing a positive relationship with his environment. He should, therefore, be given opportunity for communicating his life experiences to a sympathetic, non-manipulative listener. The latter should be able to respect the idiosyncratic limitations inherent in the cancer personality, but does not need to be a physician or psychologist.

X

The Future of the Cancer Problem

"A new scientific truth does not triumph by convincing its opponents and making them see the light, but
rather because its opponents eventually die, and a new
generation grows up that is familiar with it."

— *Max Planck*, 1949

A. *Self-Perpetuating Tendencies*

The preceding chapters have identified a number of cancerogenic
factors which are consequences of modern culture, specifically the
trend toward scientific and technological manipulation of the environment. The possibility must be considered that this trend may gain
further momentum and create a vicious circle leading toward a still
higher share of cancer as the cause of death in modern man. It is
important to realize the threatening aspects of the current situation
because there is increasing evidence that a cure may not be found by
the laboratory methods which have proved successful in the treatment
of infectious and metabolic diseases.

As far as the *biological endowment of the population* is concerned,
it must be noted that:

1. In the last century the *pool of genes* was depleted selectively

with respect to those elements which favor the symbiotic personality type. Tuberculosis tended to kill its victims before and during the reproductive period of life, whereas cancer predominates at a later period of life. Thus, the "industrial" anal type is favored genetically under present conditions.

2. *Spontaneous immunization* against neoplastic disease (Chapter V, A) has been limited by the systematic elimination of microbes from human contact.

3. *Symbiotic conditioning by natural maternal nursing* (Chapter V, B, C) *has been restricted radically* by the general practice of childbirth in hospitals and by the predominance of bottle-feeding. The first imprints on the newborn are created by inanimate objects. Searles (1960) has documented specifically that such experiences favor identification of the self and others with non-human and even with inanimate objects. [17]

4. Being genetically predisposed and experientially conditioned for the life of industrial society the *cancer-prone individuals are best suited for socio-economic success.* They are, therefore, most favored for strengthening the social influence of their mentality, and for reproducing their own kind. Concurrently, the possibilities of satisfaction and social influence become more restricted for the symbiotic personality types.

The present cultural climate provides gratification for the cancer-prone individual in many respects: a rising materialistic standard of living, activity through the expanding use of mechanical equipment, and the extension of the life span as an end in itself. It must be understood though that the modern way of life is supported not only by the cancer-prone segment of the population. The latter, so far, is only an influential minority which is most in tune with the evolutionary trend. This minority is backed up, however, by the large part of the population which is inclined to conform with the leadership of the moment (Chapter VI, B).

In view of the intricate interrelationship of biological, socio-economic and psychological factors in cancer it seems a hopeless enterprise to attack the problem by legislation and indoctrination. In this respect, the current campaigns of the English and American governments against cigarettes provide a valuable lesson. Cigarette smoking represents only a small part of the modern way of life, and its sacrifice would not interfere with any of the other "pursuits of happiness." Nevertheless, when smokers were presented authoritatively with the choice between a life without cigarettes on the one side, the risk of a premature and miserable death on the other side, the vast majority chose the latter. Their decision proves that they need the experience of individual object control so badly that they feel compelled to obtain it by symbolical behavior in addition to the available realistic forms of such satisfaction. Willingness to risk death for a particular non-vital value is certainly a reliable measure of the powerful dynamics behind the cultural system involved in the cancer epidemic. The quasi-religious dependency on cigarettes leads to the conclusion that an effective change of other modern practices cannot be expected from scientific argument and government action. The methods of infant care, the mechanization of living conditions and the commercialization of social values are deeply ingrained in contemporary culture.

B. Self-Limiting Tendencies

It would be unrealistic to conclude from the current self-perpetuating trend of the cancer epidemic that the disease will spread forever. The biology and sociology of cancer involve many consequences which are likely eventually to counteract the pathogenic factors. It may be remembered that in its early stages, the Industrial Revolution caused the spreading of tuberculosis; its consequences, however, helped to reduce the "white plague" to a very minor epidemiologic role (Dubos, 1952).

As far as the *genetic predisposition of the population* is concerned, several factors have emerged which are likely to limit selectively the reproduction of strongly cancer-prone individuals. These factors are all consequences of pregenital fixations which modern living conditions are likely to create in genetically predisposed individuals.

1. Malignancies are becoming increasingly frequent before the procreative age has been reached. Only 20 years ago they did not even figure among the 10 most frequent causes of *death in childhood.* Since then, they have become "the third greatest cause... from one to four years of age, ... and the second foremost cause ... between five and fourteen years, being exceeded only by accidents" (Ariel and Pack, 1960). We know from the thorough research of Greene (1958, 1959) that narcissistic mothers play a key role in the pathogenesis of these cases.

2. Children, particularly females, of pregenitally fixated mothers tend to *destroy their own children* when they

become parents. The growing frequency of the "battered child" syndrome suggests a defense mechanism against the danger of raising more and more maladjusted generations by means of dehumanized techniques.

3. Strongly pregenital personalities tend to *exclude themselves from procreation.* The dominant need for experiencing their powers over inanimate objects predisposes them toward reckless driving and dangerous sports with or without alcoholic complications. Furthermore, their sexual incompetence favors a homosexual way of life. Since the latter has become socially more and more accepted, such persons are less likely than formerly to marry and produce children as "proof" of sexual normality.

In considering the genetic aspects of the cancer epidemic it must also be remembered that only 15 percent of the present population is so strongly cancer-prone that it is the cause of death. Half the population dies of cardio-vascular conditions, evidence that it is predominantly social conformist (see Chapter VI, B). Thus they support the anal value system of the contemporary industrial culture, but without strong psychobiological commitment. If and when a new value system asserts itself against the present anal orientation of society, the conformist half of the population may be expected to accept and support the change.

There are reasons to expect that, in addition to genetic factors, *a change in the cultural climate* would lead to a limitation of the cancer epidemic. Again, the rising cigarette consumption may be considered. It provides evidence that the *Industrial Revolution created increasing frustrations for the anal personality type* which carried it to its stunning successes. Although the need for individualistic control is satisfied more and more in sphere of financial rewards, mechanization of work and leisure, and scientific control over parts of the natural environment, the same cannot be said about the social sphere of life. Here the scope for individualistic needs is becoming more and more restricted by the consequences of industrialization. As pointed out by Gerald Piel (1964), the publisher of the *Scientific American,* "not more than 20 percent of the American labor force is now self-employed .... In fact, the ranks of the self-employed do not include the true movers and shakers of life in America today. They are employees — members of the giant bureaucracies of the 200 or so largest industrial and financial enterprises that deploy the decisive 50 percent of the assets of our economy." The occasion for his remarks was a commencement address at Albert Einstein Medical School under the title

"Physician, Heal Thy Society." Piel's alarm was caused by the observation that "the promise of self-government, held out with such generous and humane vision less than 200 years ago, had given way to decerebrated government by spinal reflex."

It is evident that bureaucratization has not stopped on the level of government and commercial enterprise, but that it has also invaded the universities and professions. Furthermore, the gain of shorter working hours has not brought about a corresponding freedom to use the long weekends and vacations. Urbanization, traffic congestion and the organization of spectator sports and television programs restrict the individualists, although the communication media keep them aware of the many possibilities of modern life. Thus, most members of modern affluent society find themselves paradoxically in the situation of the Spanish beggars of the 16th century. They are exposed to spectacles of adventure, conquest and luxury, but without a chance of becoming active participants. Thus, the majority of males and an important minority of females have become dependent on the invention of their humble predecessors, cigarettes, to fill the gap between desires and reality.

Sensitive observers anticipated the threat of emotional impoverishment already at an early stage of the Industrial Revolution. The following quotation from Goethe's correspondence with the musician Zelter is striking. The occasion for the prophecy was a report on Spontini's new opera, *Alcidor,* which had a theme we now recognize as the conflict between anal and genital drives: the magician-ruler of a golden island fights his enemies by throwing gold pieces at their heads, but in the end love triumphs over materialistic power. The opera had impressed Zelter both by its length and by the excsses of musical technique. Goethe's answer was dated June 6, 1825, shortly before the first railroad for public transportation was inaugurated in England.

> I cannot end without coming back to that overcharged music. Everything, however, nowadays is ultra, everything transcends irresistibly in thought and in action. Nobody knows himself anymore, nobody comprehends the element in which he floats and acts, nobody the material on which he works. One cannot speak of pure simplicity, but lots of simpletons' stuff is around. Young people are stirred up much too early, and carried away in the current of the times. *Wealth* and *speed* are what the world admires and what everybody pursues. Railroads, express mail, steamboats and *all possible facilities of communication* [my italics]

are what the educated world goes in for to over-educate themselves and thus to stay in mediocrity. And this is the result of universality, that a mediocre culture becomes universal, this is the goal of the Bible Societies, of Lancaster's teaching method [the forerunner of public schools] and whatever else. Properly speaking, this is the century for the clever minds, for people with a quick grasp of what is practical. Endowed with a certain ability, they feel their superiority over the crowd although they themselves are not endowed for the highest achievements. Let us as far as possible hold on to the spirit in which we grew up; we will be, with perhaps a few others, the last of an epoch which will not return very soon. (1825)

It was part of Goethe's wisdom that he did not propose a solution for the developing impasse of cultural evolution. Many expressed similar apprehension about the future, but neither the sermons of the preachers nor the critiques of philosophers could change the course of events. It was rather the unchecked advance of materialistic science which seems to be bringing about a new value system.

C. The Reassertion of Symbiotic Values

It is apparent that the triumph of physical science over the defenses of the atom contributed to the motivations to reorganize our value system. Usually fear of the thermonuclear bomb is uppermost in people's minds. As Margaret Mead put it (1964), the new weapon established for all of mankind the social dynamics which originally had governed preliterate tribal life. There, although varied in detail, the need for group survival took precedence over the interests of the individual; but in return, the individual was protected by the group. "Today it is necessary for us to make the (social) invention that will protect every member of the human species with the sanctions that once stretched no farther than a stone could be thrown."

This goal is being implemented by another accomplishment of science, the electronic communication media. As McLuhan (1964) pointed out, television is reestablishing on a world-wide scale the immediacy of sensory contact and the shared pool of experience which safeguards the social cohesion of preliterate tribes probably even more reliably than fear of outsiders. McLuhan makes a persuasive case for the thesis that a close relationship existed between the process of individual and collective alienation of people on the one side, the development of written communication, on the other side. The latter, unlike direct speech, is not only devoid of the expressive qualifications of sound and sight, but also allows for tendentious abstractions from the integral human situation. The extension of communication beyond the range of sensual contact between sender and recipient became an essential part of the process which replaced city states with far-flung empires. The relationship between writing and aggression was envisioned in the Greek legend of King Cadmus, reputed to have invented phonetic writing, and also to have sown dragons' teeth from which sprang armed men.

It appears to be a fortunate coincidence that technology has provided the means for strengthening the potential for symbiotic behavior at the moment of history when danger of uncontrolled hostility and panic behavior has become particularly great. The phenomenon has its parallel in the development of modern psychotherapy, from classical psychoanalysis to group therapy. Freud had introduced the method of limiting the therapeutic communication severely by restricting the patient to verbal exchange with the analyst because he could not stand being stared at all day long. This is consistent with the need for unilateral relationships characteristic of cancer patients. Freud did not consider the couch *essential.* That it was taken over, nevertheless, by his whole school demonstrates that unilateral, limited communication satisfied the prevailing psychological attitude of the period. The last twenty-five years have brought about a remarkable change, inasmuch as many psychoanalysts have turned to group therapy as a frequently more effective form of treatment. It appears to be an essential element of the new procedure that full mutuality of sensory communication between therapist and patients is involved; furthermore, the therapist exposes himself to the combined scrutiny of the group.

The growing awareness of symbiotic values in human society has support in the changing emphasis of biological research. Darwin, living in the age of uncontrolled commercial competition, saw evolution nearly exclusively in terms of competitive struggle for survival, of the selective breeding of individuals most "fit" on account of superior powers of offense or defense. Forty-three years passed before the one-sided view of "nature raw in tooth and claw" was challenged by an observer from a very different cultural background. Peter Kropotkin (1902), the author of *Mutual Aid, a Factor in Evolution,* has the advantage of growing up far from the commercial and individualistic milieu of English Protestantism. Born a Russian Orthodox prince, he became sensitive to the social concern of his religion, like Tolstoy, but far more radical in his revolutionary conclusions. His contemporaries paid little attention to the zoological observations which gave biological background to his humanistic gospel, but following the catastrophe of World War I, the symbiotic aspects of animal life became rapidly an important topic of research (Portmann, 1956, 1961, 1962). Evidence has accumulated steadily that animal survival is secured to a formerly unsuspected extent by instinctual cooperation among members of the species. The diminishing importance of aggression is illustrated clearly by the observations which prove that fighting behavior is often limited to ritualized expression and becomes part of a peaceful communication system (Tinbergen, 1955; Lorenz, 1966).

Mankind had improved the animal methods of securing mutual aid by developing language, art and the technology of the communication media. The expansion of the latter suggests that the human species is undergoing an evolutionary change analogous to the transformation of instinctual behavior in animals. After 3,000 years of aggressive expansion, Western man seems to be approaching a stage of greater concern with sociability. During the periods of the Roman Empire and of Christian expansion, the community values of agricultural society had been a persistent element of internal stability because they were basic to the survival needs of the majority. As individuals became participants in the process of industrialization, their survival became dependent on a competitive power struggle. Capitalists and industrialists matched their minds; laborers, the strength and endurance of their bodies. In the jungles of the factory districts the weak were doomed to die, illustrating the principle of "natural selection." The drift toward bloody revolutions seemed inevitable until—to the surprise of Marxist theoreticians—the explosion of industrial man over the globe ended in a social implosion. Technology disposed of survival needs as a vital social problem, and the communication media are reducing rapidly the separation between nations and classes.

At the present time it seems evident that survival needs are no longer a vital problem and that labor and management are learning to distribute the growing national wealth by peaceful methods. As the hierarchies of government, of labor and of capital become more alike and even interchangeable, the standard of living for the strong and for the weak becomes more alike for the majority of the population. The right to a livelihood for the unemployed is no longer seriously questioned by any party. The new social order resembles the pecking order of the poultry yard where the relative dominance of individual members of the group is established without destructive power contests.

The evolution of a controlling community spirit is highlighted by the fact that economists have begun to discuss the possibility of a guaranteed income for every citizen (Reagan, 1964; Theobald, 1965). Although this may never happen exactly in the form suggested, the underlying socio-economic condition can hardly be questioned. There is a diminishing motivation for economic competition. At the same time, the controlling influence of the state in all economic activities limits for most people the prospects of exercising much control over their economic affairs. In psychoanalytical terms this means that anal motivations are reduced for the average conformist person as far as social inducements are concerned. Obviously there will always be those who are strongly motivated by genetic endowment and infantile conditioning to create an anal way of life.

The changing character of the industrial civilization suggests analogies to previous cultural attainments of mankind. Neither the primitive hunters nor planters could have conquered their specific realms of nature without strong motivation for unilateral object control. They, like the participants in the Industrial Revolution, must have acquired their technical skills and social structures under ascetic conditions and by raw methods of aggression. Once the material foundations of culture had been acquired, more complex levels of social organization, of religion, arts and sciences developed in many races and regions. One may expect higher humanistic developments from industrial civilization because it is in the process of transferring mechanical labor to machines. In previous high cultures the leisure and the economic means for creative accomplishments had always been provided by the exploitation of the underprivileged fellow human beings. Now, for the first time in the history of mankind, mechanical labor is being transferred increasingly to machinery and for all citizens a certain amount of non-utilitarian experience and activity is becoming available. It is evident that these opportunities are being used widely, even though often in socially and spiritually disturbing ways. Alcoholism, drug addiction and much of what the entertainment industry offers, however, cannot be held up legitimately as examples of a decline of Western civilization from the level of earlier Christian ages. Those also had their dark aspects, and many of the illnesses of our own age can be traced to the all-too-confident virtues of its predecessors.

Positive aspects of the changing cultural climate are particularly evident in the *growing popularity of art and literature,* both as a vocation and as a market commodity. Seen from the psychoanalytical point of view the production of utilitarian goods and of art are equally derived from the dynamics of the anal instinct, but seen from the social point of view, there is a significant difference. Utilitarian activities are motivated by *individual survival needs,* they are therefore essentially asocial, and, when threatened, lead to behavior like that of a struggle for survival. Artistic activities, on the other hand, are motivated chiefly by *social needs.* A work of art has reality to the extent to which it achieves communication between its author and the public. This basic social value is present even if the public is limited to one person, and even if the aesthetic and spiritual value is of a low order. As long as an experience is *shared* is affirms symbiotic values. In psychoanalytical parlance the anal function is subordinated to the genital level of functioning. Even the artist who is willing to prostitute his endowment for utilitarian purposes can do so only to the extent to which he meets the needs of his customers.

It seems unnecessary to document the fact that the American scene has changed radically since 1925 when Calvin Coolidge asserted "The business of America is business." Business building and factories, not so long ago expressions of pure utilitarianism, aspire more and more to provide aesthetic satisfaction as well, private homes are becoming pervaded with the sights and sounds of the works of living and dead artists. At the same time the private lives of the population give evidence that genital dynamics assert themselves not only through the medium of the arts, but also in the emphasis on communication through sexual intercourse.

In a preceding chapter (VII, B, C) it was made clear that the Industrial Revolution and the scientific "conquest of nature" have caused a deep and widespread disturbance in the capacity for spontaneous physical relationships between men and women. The consequences were noticeable not only in the sphere of modern love life, but in the distortion of social relationships by fixation on the anal level—apt to favor the development of cancer.

Modern scientific developments have begun to implement effectively the popular instinct which asserts the importance of the sexual sphere, not only on the level of maturity, but also on the level of its infantile foundations. After the nearly exclusively clinical approach to labor and infant-feeding in the beginning of this century, a trend toward "natural childbirth" and breast-feeding is developing. Simultaneously, medicine has found ways to separate the affectional intention of intercourse from unintentional procreation. In the face of the population explosion, contraception is necessary to save the natural association of sex and love from the destructive effect of practical and moralistic inhibitions. The dynamics of the cancer epidemic teach the same lesson: that in order to reduce its *social* causes, the priority of affection over fertility must be recognized by the law and the moralists. Even the Roman Catholic Church has weakened her stand. In a symposium on "Sexuality and the Modern World" Father DeLestapis, S.J. (1964) spelled out what psychoanalysis suggests, that the foundation of marriage rests on "greater intersubjectivity of the conjugal dialogue" and that children will benefit from the emotional improvement of the marital relationship. He agrees with Jean Guitton that "Love, the oldest of subjects, can also be the newest... It has some chance by the upcoming generation because the application of knowledge to love, which has been a cause of darkness, can also be the cause of light."

It is apparent that the current evolution of industrialized nations is leading up to a new collective spirit of culture. On the levels of technology and psychotherapy, biological understanding and social organization, in the appreciation of receptive pleasure, aesthetics and sex, the consequences favor an overcoming of the conditions which created the original causes of the cancer epidemic. In psychoanalytical terms, the excessive development of anal values leads to a crisis, cancer, with two possible outcomes: death, or, recovery if a re-assertion of genital values occurs. It is interesting to note that the essence of this drama was originally told in the Old Testament and it was interpreted at the beginning of the Industrial Revolution by William Blake through his illustrations of the Book of Job (Blake, 1935; Hagstrum, 1964). It was the same year Goethe commented so pessimistically on the beginning of the age of the railroad.

Job is shown first as "the wealthiest man of all the East," the embodiment of the Puritan capitalist "who fears God and turns away from evil." He observes a bleak "English Sunday" in prayer with his family while musical instruments hang unused from a tree. The end of this phase comes with the loss of all his possessions and children. Job himself contracts a loathsome disease covering his whole body. His salvation comes as God reveals to him His creativity in nature. He begets as many children as he had before and with them, transcends the barren morality of his former life, communing with God through music, the least material of the arts. The biblical text contains only one cue from which Blake developed his concept that Job was converted to art, the statement that his second lot of daughters was "most beautiful" and that the patriarch gave them equal inheritance with his sons. The parallel between the afflictions of Job and the perils of modern man appears as striking as his salvation through a new understanding of nature and art. Anticipating the developments of the 20th century, the conversion of Job even includes recognition of the equality of the sexes, departing from the old social order.

C. Cancer Prophylaxis

Spontaneous changes in our industrial culture encourage the expectation that the cancerogenic influences affecting the present population will be reduced. The question arises whether deliberate prophylactic measures could speed up the self-healing process..

As pointed out previously, the logical place to begin a program of change would be at birth by indoctrinating mothers on the emotional needs of their babies and encouraging breast feeding. The effects of such teachings, however, are limited by the fact that so many mothers have been emotionally warped by their own infantile experiences that they cannot participate successfully in such a program. Often too, there is an additional complication arising when husbands are jealous of the intimacy between their wives and children.

Theoretically, the next best step would be to identify by psychological testing the cancer-prone individuals and to give them guidance with respect to the specific requirements of their individual life situations, analogous to the procedure suggested for patients who already have been treated for cancer (Chapter IX). It would not be too difficult to implement a medical check-up with a Rorschach test since the administration and scanning for cancer criteria take rarely more than 20-30 minutes. In all likelihood a psychologist could design a specific perception test using a simplified version of the tendencies abstracted from the Rorschach findings (Chapter II, B).

Practically speaking, the spotting of cancer-prone individuals would be desirable only in the cases where exposure to known carcinogens is contemplated, e.g., work processing nickel, chrome and uranium. As discussed previously, in the case of cigarette smoking, the proportion between the carcinogenic and the tranquilizing factors is not clearly established (Chapter VIII, B-3). It is questionable, however, that a systematic search for cancer-prone individuals would produce good results. On the one hand, medicine has not developed the wisdom and insights which would entitle it to offer psycho-social guidance to a person who does not feel the need for it. Often enough, even those who seek help from psychiatrists, psychologists and social workers receive the kind of guidance which causes more trouble. Then there is a specific handicap inherent in the cancer-prone personality, that he resists communication and guidance. Even those who are manifestly threatened by the experience of actual cancer are reluctant to abandon their old ways merely for the sake of prolonging their lives. It has been noted that chronic cancer worriers are often most negligent in dealing with beginning cancer symptoms. Thus, under present conditions, screening for potential cancer patients would be apt to increase the number of phobias without decreasing the incidence of the disease.

The qualification "under present conditions" was used advisedly because the prevailing medical attitude toward cancer treats the patient in a way which is most incompatible with his psychological needs. He needs a sense of personal control over his body and way of life, whereas physicians concentrate on controlling the "invading tumor" and consider the patient himself as the passive victim, rather than a participating personality. It is understandable that cancer-prone personalities are intuitively averse to this situation and that, therefore, a major prophylactic task is to bring about a change in the therapeutic atmosphere.

Evans (1926) formulated a psychosocial approach to cancer over 40 years ago,[18] but it has encountered strong resistance for two main reasons.

1. The great successes of modern medicine were based on a theoretical model of the organism which was applied to protozoan and man alike. It was defined as a physico-chemical mechanism engaged in the transformation of energy, and controllable by judicious physico-chemical methods on the level of cell metabolism as well as on the level of specific brain functions.

   The cancer epidemic demonstrates that the physico-chemical manipulation of human life is apt to frustrate vital symbiotic needs. The neoplastic process marks the point at which the old way of thinking does not provide a viable existence. The new way recognizes that life is based on mutual transactions between two or more living organisms, on field phenomena, rather than on complex physico-chemical reactions.

   Radical changes of a theoretical concept are reluctantly accepted by the scientific community if the old one has been satisfactory for a long enough time. Even in as impersonal a discipline as physics, the replacement of the Newtonian theories by those of Einstein and Planck encountered irrational resistance. As Planck put it in his *Scientific Auto-biography:* "A new scientific truth does not triumph by convincing its opponents and making them see the light, but rather because its opponents eventually die, and a new generation grows up that is familiar with it."

2. In the field of medicine the problem of a fundamental *change of thought is made more difficult because it directly affects the health and livelihood of so many people.* In the face of a dangerous disease it is very difficult to abandon a rationale which has cured many other diseases. Fear does not favor thinking, but rather a regression to infantile behavior and clinging to old habits of thought. This reaction is re-enforced by the fact that socio-economic interests are often behind mechanistically oriented medical research. It is hardly an accident that one of the most important of this type of research center for cancer, the Sloan-Kettering Institute in New York, bears the names of two General Motors executives, and that the cigarette industry established the first academic chair for parapsychology, the most unsomatic form of interpersonal communication, at Duke University.

The preceding observations on the distorting effect of socio-economic interests on medicine are not related only to the cancer problem. The Committee on Science in the Promotion of Human Welfare (American Association for the Advancement of Science) stated on more general grounds that "there is some evidence that the integrity of science is beginning to erode under the abrasive pressure of its close partnership with economic, social and political affairs" (Rosenblith, 1961).

The psychosocial aspects of cancer are at the core of the more diffuse manifestations of the conflict between mechanistic and truly biological medicine. Recognition of the psychosomatic character of this disease would therefore imply a major break-through for the next revolution in medicine, a renaissance of humanism (Kruse, 1964). There are hopeful signs that the general public interest in "the whole person" and the specialized application to neoplastic processes will mutually reinforce each other and improve the conditions of therapy for the patients of the future.

E. Conclusion

Understanding the individual patient is helped by seeing him in the context of the collective forces which provided the constellation for the epidemic frequency of the disease. The contemporary emphasis on individual independence, material needs and unilateral control of some physical area of the world is reflected even in personalities whose concern is with the mind rather than the body; for instance, Freud's materialistic concept of the psyche, or Wittgenstein's philosophy of language, or Pope John XXIII's concrete approach to the ecumenical movement. The most general dominator of the industrial age and its cancerogenic implications is the phrase "man's conquest of nature."

Seen in its cultural context, cancer loses the character of a physical demon invading human bodies and demanding scientific exorcism through the machinery of physical science. Each tumor appears as a symptom of a losing existential encounter between the world and a person predominantly identified with the spirit of the industrial age. The encounter either ends in death or in a changed relationship between the patient and his environment. Thus nothing can be accomplished by campaigns for the "conquest of cancer." The expression itself is a reminder that the human problem of the cancer patient is ignored.

A realistic attitude regarding the cancer problem calls for the philosophy developed by Freud's less heroic but wiser disciple, Jung. He showed himself to be, in the form of his death, a vascular type and thus was emotionally uninvolved in the issue. From this point of view he wrote: "The greatest and most important problems of life...can never be solved, but only outgrown." By this he meant a "raising of the level of consciousness through which the insoluble problem loses its urgency. It is not solved logically in its own terms, but fades out in contrast to a new and stronger life tendency."

The insoluble problem of cancer is the polarity between two basic life forces:

1. the evolutionary, creative potential of nature and the human spirit;
2. the static hereditary limitations of physical forms.

There are indications that the "conquest of nature" is fading out as the supreme goal of human endeavor. What seems to be growing is the awareness of the healing which comes from conscious participation in the life of nature.

Appendix

Common Gestalt Tendencies of Prehistoric Art and of Rorschach Percepts

The stability of the two genetic psychobiological orientations is illustrated by the persistence of the same specific gestalt tendencies in prehistoric art forms and in contemporary perception of Rorschach's inkblots. This phenomenon provides a concrete background for understanding diseases as the product of specific affinities between constitution and environment, an understanding which is necessary for understanding the origin of the cancer epidemic.

PREHISTORIC ART

A. *Hunters*

1. Single figures and scenes are placed on the cave walls without concern for their aesthetic inter-relationships. Every artistic act and its subject matter express concentration on an immediate purpose, without concern for the total situation.

2. Human and animal actions are pictures.

3. Pointed tools, weapons and phalluses are typical moveable artifacts.

B. *Planters*

1. Round vessels provide the foundation for ornamentation with balanced, static geometrical and natural forms. They express the orderly pattern of the recurrent seasons of plant life.

RORSCHACH PERCEPTION

A. *L Group*

1. Solitary human and animal figures are perceived in the central part of the inkblots.

2. Kinesthesis predominantly expresses goal-directed actions.

3. The same objects prevail over non-aggressive objects in the central part of the inkblots.

B. *V Group*

1. The symmetrical halves of the inkblot are perceived as two human beings or animals in a balanced mutual relationship.

2. Human and animal figures are static.

2. Human and animal figures are either static or kinesthesis expresses activities determined by social convention.

3. The artifact is hollow.

3. The central part tends to be interpreted as an opening (sometimes a flower or vagina), as unstructured (water, fire) or as a ritualistic object (totempole, mace, cross).

There is another specific difference between the Rorschach perceptions of the L and the V group which has no direct counterpart in the prehistoric art works, but confirms the pervasiveness of the two specific life styles on the perception of the environment. This difference is expressed in the preference for seeing certain animals.

L Group

V Group

a) The *eagle*, the old symbol of individual freedom and power.

a) Cattle and sheep represent collective, domesticated life. Experimental neurosis of sheep takes the form of cardiovascular symptom (Liddell, 1942).

b) The *pig*, in keeping with the "pigheadedness" of this group. Liddel (1942) demonstrated that experimental neurosis in this animal takes the form of violent motor activities.

Beasts of prey symbolize destructive tendencies. They are far more frequent in the Rorschach responses of the cardiovascular than of the locomotor group (chi-square 28.041, p 0.01). In my original publication (1946) I left this difference uninterpreted because I lacked clinical and anthropological insight into what seemed to me a paradoxical finding. At the present time the finding appears consistent with the different attitudes of the two groups toward the value of fellow human beings and animals:

Locomotor Group

The individual is highly valued. Primitive hunters believe that man and animal survive death as spirits which in case of slayings must be propitiated. Killing of animals is incidental to survival needs, human sacrifice does not exist. The aggression of arthritis and Parkinson patients is confined to the assertion of individual ego ideals, a confinement which finds concrete expression in the restriction of the locomotor functions when the individual encounters overwhelming resistance from the environment and becomes sick.

Cardiovascular Group

The group is valued more highly than the individual. Primitive planters identify man and animal with their plants which must die in order to give rise to new generations of men, animals and plants. Ritualistic sacrifices of individuals therefore are used to insure magically the survival of tribe, flocks and crops. The aggression of cardiovascular patients is more powerfully developed because their actions are dictated by the group which demands conformity and the sacrifice of individualistic ideals. They die when they cannot live according to the expectations of their social environment. The Biblical story of the first murder is psychologically correct: Cain, the planter, kills his brother, enraged that God approved of Abel's animal sacrifice, but not of his own sacrifice of seeds.

TABLE I

Frequencies of Rorschach Criteria
for Cancer and Tuberculosis

Clinical Groups	N.	Total Figures for Groups Criteria				Individual Variations Criteria			Means		
		Resp.	Ca	TB	Ratio	Resp.	Ca	TB	R	Ca	TB
Lung Cancer	26	543	330	123	1:0.37	7-60	7-15	1- 8	20.8	12.8	4.7
Other Cancers*	67	1539	749	353	1:0.47	6-93	3-20	0-13	22.9	10.9	5.2
Art. Hypertension	60	1565	528	423	1:0.81	5-94	3-15	1-15	26.1	8.8	7.5
Pulm. Tuberculosis	82	1505	416	949	1:2.28	6-61	0-13	3-20	18.3	5.1	11.5
TOTALS:	235					5-94	0-20	0-20			
*Groups: Cervix	38	767	416	189	1:0.30	9-93	3-20	0-11			
Breast	7	246	97	53	1:0.57	15-71	8-18	1-13			
Oral-Anal	10	203	107	52	1:0.49	10-45	5-17	2-13			
Melanoma	3	45	24	6	1:0.25	6-27	5- 9	1- 4			
Liver	2	96	26	11	1:0.42	20-76	13	3- 8			
Hodgkins	1	18	13	3	1:0.23	18	13	3			
Gonads	6	164	66	39	1:0.59	10-75	5-17	2-12			

TABLE II

Frequencies of Cancer and Tuberculosis Criteria
for Individual Plates and for Total Score of Plates

Clinical Diagnosis	Rorschach Criteria	I	II	III	IV	V	VI	VII	VIII	IX	X	Totals	Positive Cases (%)
Lung Cancer N=26	Ca	32	39	52	49	6	29	16	42	21	44	330	100
	TB	14	15	24	16	1	8	6	18	5	16	123	—
Other Cancers N=67	Ca	63	86	105	131	16	80	43	87	40	88	749	95.5
	TB	28	36	44	34	12	26	17	49	33	74	353	4.5
Arterial Hypertension N=60	Ca	27	83	90	83	11	51	34	69	24	56	528	65
	TB	29	30	63	55	13	41	28	57	29	78	423	20
	None												15
Pulmonary Tuberculosis N=82	Ca	23	57	53	57	11	45	14	57	24	73	413	9.8
	TB	58	113	155	122	28	64	65	127	71	125	935	87.7
	None												3.5

TABLE III

Results of Rorschach Diagnosis for Individual Plates and for Total Score of Plates

Clinical Diagnosis	Rorschach Diagnosis	I	II	III	IV	V	VI	VII	VIII	IX	X	Diagnostic Balance	All Plates (%)
Lung Cancer N=26	Ca	12	17	20	19	6	18	16	19	15	16	26	100
	TB	1	2	3	2	1	1	4	4	2	5	—	—
	Neither	13	7	3	5	19	7	6	3	9	5	—	—
Other Cancers N=67	Ca	32	42	43	48	13	54	42	41	26	30	65	97
	TB	11	3	13	4	9	3	15	14	18	14	2	3
	Neither	24	22	11	15	45	10	10	12	23	23	—	—
Arterial Hypertension N=60	Ca	11	39	29	31	8	23	31	24	14	9	36	60
	TB	17	8	15	16	10	9	23	17	14	20	10	17
	Neither	32	13	16	13	42	28	6	19	32	31	14	23
Pulmonary Tuberculosis N=82	Ca	10	14	9	18	8	21	4	16	10	24	8	7.3
	TB	32	49	52	52	25	22	45	47	48	39	74	92.7
	Neither	40	19	21	12	49	39	33	39	24	19	—	—

TABLE IV

Frequencies of Specific and Unspecific Percepts

Number	Diagnosis	Total Percepts	Minus	Critical Percepts	Equals	Unspecific Percepts	%
26	Lung cancer	543	-	453	=	90	17
67	Other cancers	1539	-	1102	=	437	32
60	Arterial hypertension	1565	-	951	=	614	39
82	Tuberculosis	1505	-	1365	=	140	9

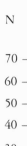

CANCER (N = 93)

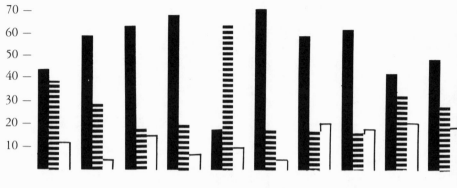

TUBERCULOSIS (N = 82)

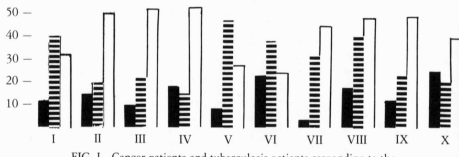

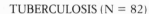

FIG. I   Cancer patients and tuberculosis patients responding to the
individual Rorschach cards   according to cancer type   ■

neutral   ≡

according to tuberculosis type □

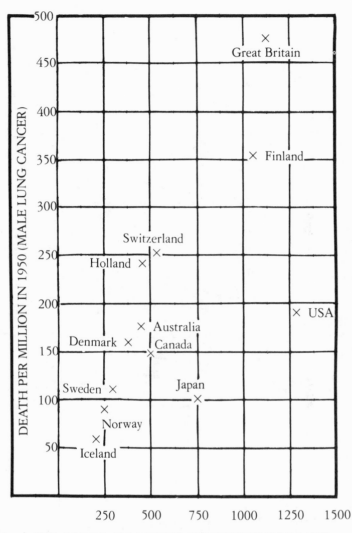

FIG. II (see page 186) Cigarette consumption in 1930 and incidence of male lung cancer in 1950. All figures are according to Doll (1955) with the exception of the figures for Japan (Todd. 1959).

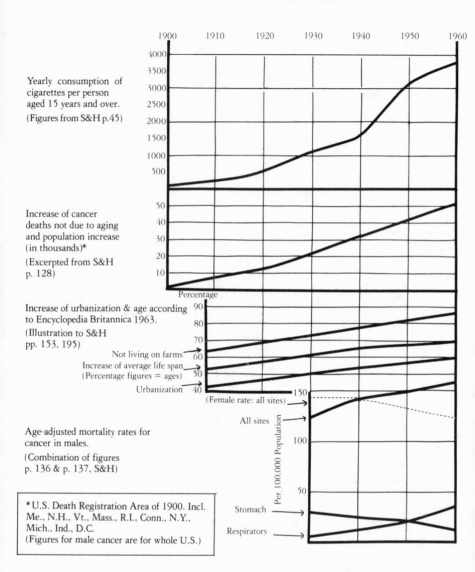

1900   1910   1920   1930   1940   1950   1960

Yearly consumption of cigarettes per person aged 15 years and over.
(Figures from S&H p.45)

Increase of cancer deaths not due to aging and population increase (in thousands)*
(Excerpted from S&H p. 128)

Increase of urbanization & age according to Encyclopedia Britannica 1963.
(Illustration to S&H pp. 153, 195)

Not living on farms →
Increase of average life span →
(Percentage figures = ages)
Urbanization →

(Female rate: all sites) →

All sites →

Age-adjusted mortality rates for cancer in males.
(Combination of figures p. 136 & p. 137, S&H)

Per 100,000 Population

Stomach →
Respiratory →

*U.S. Death Registration Area of 1900. Incl. Me., N.H., Vt., Mass., R.I., Conn., N.Y., Mich., Ind., D.C.
(Figures for male cancer are for whole U.S.)

FIG. III   Parallel trends of increase in cancer, specifically male cancer and lung cancer, in urbanization and in cigarette consumption (p. 196).
(S&H = *Smoking and Health, Report of the Advisory Committee to the Surgeon General of the Public Health Service,* Washington, 1964)

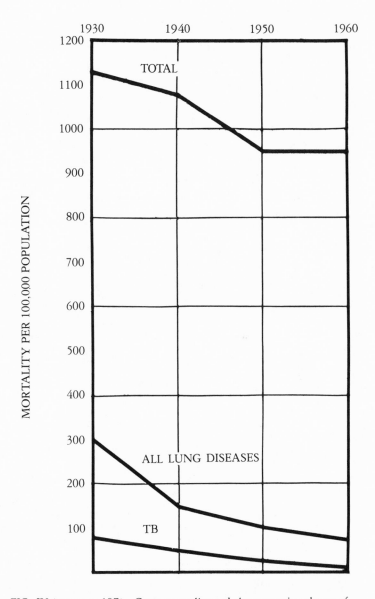

FIG. IV (see page 197)   Gross mortality and the respective shares of tuberculosis and of all lung disease (tuberculosis, cancer and pneumonia) from 1930 until 1960.

U.S. Public Health Service Vital Statistics

Notes

1   The possibility must be considered that a *DNA fragment of the tuber-culosis bacterium* may be involved in cancerogenesis. This hypothesis is suggested by the fact that Harlow's Rhesus monkeys never developed neoplasias, even though this is a disease liability of the species, and even though the experiments with "motherless monkeys" created conditions that were analogous to Greene's (1958, 1959) observations of leukemia associated with deprivation of maternal affection. Harlow informed me that his entire colony is daily fed a small amount of isoniazid because the species is extremely tuberculosis-prone, and that consequently there has not been a single case of tuberculosis. Harlow assumed that the absence of neoplasia has been due to the fact that his monkeys had not reached "cancer age," but he ignored the high incidence of leukemia in human children. My own hypothesis assumes that the exclusion of tuberculosis also involved the exclusion of cancerogenic DNA. Salk (1971) considered this hypothesis interesting and regretted that his commitments did not allow him to evaluate it experimentally.

2   Most practitioners of the "classical" Rorschach method (cf. pg. I-10 and ff.) are not likely to be interested in a fundamentally new approach. As Max Planck observed with regard to quantum physics: "A new scientific truth does not triumph by convincing its opponents and making them see the light, but rather because its opponents eventually die, and a new generation grows up that is familiar with it."

3   Fear of involuntary self-revelation may be one of the reasons why psychiatrists have generally avoided the Rorschach method, and why psychologists have tended to interpret records in abstract terms and in "Rorschachese" language. Tosquelles (1945) observed that, even without being given interpretations, people realized as an afterthought that they had exposed unintentionally things about themselves which they had been used to concealing. He mentioned that in the last war he had reason to regret that he showed the cards to some of his military superiors, although he had not given them any interpretations of their reactions after they had asked for a look to satisfy their curiosity. Even professional familiarity with the inkblots does not counteract this hypnotic effect. Many experts who consulted me on account of their personal problems surprised themselves by their own percepts when I administered the plates to them.

4   It is necessary to remind the reader that control studies require know-

ledge of the findings of the original investigator. In 1951 Prichard, Schwab and Tillman claimed that the Rorschach records of their Parkinson cases did not show any common personality traits, contrary to my own findings (Booth 1946a, 1946b, 1948). At my request, the psychologist in charge of the testing sent me the original Rorschach records, which confirmed my original claims. The psychologist explained that he had not been told about my work and therefore had been unable to check his records in respect of the criteria I had defined. He had been put in the situation of a student who would be asked to find what the blood specimens of 10 persons of blood group A has in common, before having learned of the existence of blood groups.

5

AGE RANGE	CA (n 15)	TB (n 35)
25-40	3	7
41-50	4	10
51-60	2	16
61-70	6	2
MEDIAN AGE	53	49

6 The so-called "Birth of Venus" in the National Museum of Rome originally formed one wing of a large altar, the other wing of which is now in the Museum of Fine Arts in Boston and plausibly named "The Contest of Aphrodite and Persephone." That the catalogue of the Boston museum nevertheless refers to the relief in Rome by its mistaken title, is one of the numerous examples of imperceptive descriptions of many works of art in museum catalogues on which the great art historian, Heinrich Woelfflin, commented in 1907 ("Ueber Galeriekataloge" in "Kleine Schriften 1886-1933" Basel, Schwabe, 1946).

7 Women who have not been breast fed often lack adequate instinctual capacity for fulfilling the emotional and instinctual needs of dyadic nursing. There are enough instances in which women fulfill only the nutritional purpose, and in this case the consequences for the infant are likely to be worse than those of bottle feeding. As Newton and Newton asserted (1967), medical encouragement of breast feeding should be supported by routine rooming-in of the baby with the mother. The current custom of separating them at birth except for brief feeding times provides too little opportunity for the development of the spontaneous dyadic relationship of which nursing is a much

overrated part. Actually, some mothers with neurotic breast problems are interacting more freely with their babies while giving them the bottle than while forcing themselves to breast-feed.

8 Many physicians and psychologists are so strongly prejudiced against a psychodynamic concept of any disease with somatic pathology that they unconsciously forget to ask relevant psychological questions. Some years ago, I had a chance to observe this phenomenon in the case of Parkinsonism. A neurosurgeon had tried to interest a clinical psychologist on his staff in my psychodynamic approach (Booth, 1948). The psychologist read my paper and invited me to sit in on his interviews of candidates for subcortical surgery. After he had finished,he invited me to ask my own questions. In every instance we found that the psychologist had forgotten to ask the relevant question. When I asked the patient, he readily answered with information that verified my expectations. The psychologist was sufficiently impressed to plan a systematic control study after my summer vacation, but nothing came of it. Evidently, the Department felt as threatened as the cancer departments that I approached in 1942 with the request to let me administer Rorschach tests to their patients (Booth, 1965).

9 The conformism of the cardiovascular type cannot be explained as a consequence of either socio-economic insecurity or lack of intellectual understanding. Resistance to my unconventional psychobiological research came from three later victims of cardiovascular disease who definitely were not limited by such problems.

   In 1942, I submitted the project of my Rorschach study of cancer to Dr. C. P. Rhoads, at that time director of the Sloan-Kettering Institute for Cancer Research. He studied it, found it sound, and promised to arrange for my access to patients. When I asked him a few weeks later, however, he ignored a number of written and telephonic inquiries. (I may add that the project was financially funded by an outside sponsor.) I finally asked Dr. Carl Binger, who had introduced me to Dr. Rhoads, what had happened. The answer was that nothing had changed his favorable opinion of my project and of my person, but that he had thought of the likelihood that the Board of Trustees would find out that he considered the possibility of a psychological factor in cancer. He was afraid that the Board would no longer trust his judgment and would cut off the funds on which the Institute depended.

   Many years later, Dr. Smiley Blanton, a friend of Alfred Sloan, who was then chairman of General Motors and trustee of the Institute, told me that Sloan had confidentially said to him: "Personally, I am convinced that a spiritual problem is involved in cancer, and I would love to support research dealing with it. But I can't, because if any of my business associates would find out about it, they would think that I am off my rocker and no longer trust my judgment in business matters."

In 1952 I asked Dr. Binger, now Editor-in-Chief of *Psychosomatic Medicine*, why he had accepted the negative opinions of two readers to whom he had given a paper I had submitted for publication. His answer was: "Psychosomatic medicine is still controversial and many of my colleagues consider me a romantic for espousing this cause. Your ideas are far more radical than mine, and I cannot compromise my professional standing by publishing them. Very possibly twenty years from now you will be proven right and I, wrong; but at the present time I cannot take responsibility for papers which are not acceptable at Harvard Medical School." Perhaps it is worth mentioning that this 1952 paper had nothing to do with cancer, but with another touchy psychosomatic problem. I shelved it at that time, in spite of positive reviews from other responsible colleagues, because I had just started my cancer research, thanks to the support of Dr. Nolan D.C. Lewis and Dr. Alvan Barach of the Columbia College of Physicians and Surgeons.

10   Inman (1961) has published an excellent concise account of the history of the case of breast cancer which developed in a maternity nurse. He covers the infantile background, the physical and psychological traumas of adult life, the operation of the localized tumor, the survival of multiple metastases and also implicitly the responsiveness to genuine human concern.

In the course of three interviews the observant psychoanalyst unfolded all the features of the interaction between personality and environment which have been described as typical of cancer in the course of the present monograph. The complete agreement between the empirical study of one case, and the theoretical deductions from Rorschach records is worth mentioning because there had been no communication between Inman and myself before his publication and my first attempt to publish a shorter version of my findings, both taking place in 1961.

11   Hoernecke and Berndt (1965) did not find increased familial incidence of lung cancer because they did not consider the fact that the lung is the seat of numerous competing disease processes: tuberculosis, emphysema, chronic bronchitis and asthma. The breast is liable to only one deadly disease and disease disposition of the breast is therefore identical with cancer as far as mortality statistics are concerned.

12 Closer observation of other cancer forms may reveal greater frequency of depression in the early stages than has been realized by modern physicians. The recent report of Fras and Litkin (1966) on cancer of the pancreas, and on retroperitoneal malignant lymphoma is pertinent. The fact that depression was found infrequently in cancer of the colon may be the result of the coincidence of anal infantile disposition with the anal implications of the organ disposition of the last-mentioned group. It must be remembered that in the last century eminent physicians like Sir James Paget and Willard Parker were certain that all cancer patients are depressed (Kowal, 1953).

13 Doll and Hill (1964), after a 10-year follow-up of British doctors, found that in this group the lung cancer mortality declined progressively after giving up smoking, but was still two to three times higher than among those who never had smoked. They also found the death rate much higher among inhalers than among non-inhalers. All this is consistent with the concept that the more vitally dependent people are on cigarettes, the more intensively they smoke and the earlier they die as a result of their carcinogenic tension, particularly when deprived of their tension reducer. Consequently, from year to year the original group of smokers is reduced to those who are not lung cancer prone.

14 When in the last century masturbation was considered a major cause of diseases, the suppression by outright punishment, by painful contraptions and by surgery (castration and clitoridectomy) were widely practiced in Europe and America (Spitz, 1952).

15 Those who skipped the chapter on the rationale of the Rorschach Test may be reminded that the 10 inkblots operate in the same manner as the dummies used by ethologists. One cannot perceive them except in terms of one's own dynamics, i.e., in each card those features become determinants which are most satisfactory to the instinctual needs of the percipient under the conditions provided by the given inkblot.

16 The symbolic therapeutic value of reducing surgically the cancerous organ would be consistent with the findings of Shrifte (1962). This author found that a bad prognosis is related to the amount of unused vitality in the patient. The rationale of this aspect of cancer therapy is the same as the method of "symbolic realization" developed by Sechehaye (1951) for schizophrenia.

17 The phenomenon of identification with non-human and inanimate

objects exists in preliterate societies although they are raised at the breast. The latter experience prevents, however, the disturbance of sexual functions and of symbiotic social relationships which plagues modern man.

18   A few facts may be mentioned to illustrate this statement because it may appear incredible in the present period of popular concern with psychosomatic medicine. Nevertheless, even the members of the American Psychosomatic Society showed, in 1953, so little interest in neoplastic disease that Georg Engel made the phenomenon the subject of his presidential address (Engel, 1954). This courageous effort did not have much effect. Six years later the editor of *Psychosomatic Medicine* sponsored a 24-page review of the considerable world literature on psychosomatic aspects of cancer (Perrin and Pierce, 1959). The authors arrived at the conclusion that not one of these publications satisfied their standards of scientific evidence. Their concept of science is evidently taken from the methods of studying inanimate nature and belongs to the current form of clinical research which has called forth the criticism of Sir Robert Platt quoted approvingly by H. D. Kruse (1964): "As part of its rigidity and stereotypy, clinical science tends to recognize only one kind of science. It ends... to use mostly repeatable planned scientific experimentation with controlled variables. It seeks a homogeneity of clinical material that is quite unobtainable. It neglects the method of empirical clinical observation and hypotheses to explain it. (He) believes that *controlling variables may conceal facts.*"

Considering the fact that *Psychosomatic Medicine* is a journal devoted to the study of the inseparable unity of psyche and soma, the publication of the completely negative review of the application to cancer constitutes practically a declaration that cancer is an exception, really the demonic "invader" of the autonomous psychosomatic organism. The thorough-going defensive effort against the psychological study of cancer illustrates the importance of considering this disease in the context of its cultural setting. Research and therapy are so deeply involved in the materialistic values of industrial society that any direct or implied criticsm of their rationale is experienced by most professionals as a real threat to their existence. Their subjective stake in the physicalistic methods of dealing with the cancer problem is frequently betrayed by the emotional pitch of the many rationalizations which are used in defense against those who are insisting that this disease is as psychosomatic as all manifestations of life (Booth, 1965; LeShan, 1965). Many psychosomaticists seem to sense the seriousness of the social problem and therefore restrict themselves to diseases which are not directly related to the value crisis of contemporary society. The individual and social values involved in the rheumatic, cardio-vascular and infectious diseases have been part of mankind since prehistoric times and they can be acted upon still in an industrialized and urbanized society. For these old-fashioned personality types the industrial age has only changed secondary matters, primary for all of them has always been the attitude that the world is there to be lived with, not to be conquered.

Secondly, it should be pointed out that in 1965 *Psychosomatic Medicine* reviewed a five-day international conference on the psychosomatic aspects of neoplastic disease in less than one column; the reviewer stating frankly that as a chemotherapist he was not altogether conversant with the subject matter.

Considering the scepticism in the circles of the American Psychosomatic Society it is not surprising that of the 10 members of the Surgeon General's Committee on Smoking and Health, not one is associated with psychosomatic medicine, not even one of the 189 contributors to the report. Of the latter group only 4.7 percent are identified as psychologists, not one as a psychiatrist.

Finally, it should be mentioned that the defensiveness against a psychosomatic study of cancer is not a local American problem. When in 1960 the International Psychosomatic Cancer Study Group convened for the first time, similar experiences were reported by European colleagues.

Bibliography of Gotthard Booth, M.D.

1935   "Paralysis Agitans." *Der Nervenartz* 2, 69-83.

1936a   ----- and Bruno Klopfer, "Personality Studies in Chronic Arthritis." *Rorschach Res. Exch.* 1/2 : 40-48.

1936b   "Material for a Comparative Case Study of a Chronic Arthritis Personality." *Rorschach Res. Exch.* 1/2 : 49.

1937a   "The F+ Responses." *Rorschach Res. Exch.* 2/2 : 48-53.

1937b   "Personality and Chronic Arthritis." *The Journal of Nervous and Mental Disease* 85/6, 637-662.

1937c   "The Use of Graphology in Medicine." *The Journal of Nervous and Mental Disease* 86/6, 674-679.

1939a   "The Psychological Approach in Therapy of Chronic Arthritis." *Rheumatism,* January, 1-12.

1939b   "Objective Techniques in Personality Testing." *Archives of Neurology and Psychiatry* 42, 1-17 (reprint).

1939c   "Response to Klopfer." Minutes of the 16th Annual Meeting of the American Orthopsychiatric Association: *Rorschach Res. Exch.* 3/3, 112-113.

1944   *The Church and Returning Service Personnel: No. 1 Attitudes and Problems.* Philadelphia: Committee on Camp and Church Activities of the Presbyterian War-Time Service Commission.

1945   "Psychosomatic Medicine." *Inward Light* 25, 4-7.

1946a   "Variety in Personality and Its Relation to Health." *The Review of Religion* 10, 385-412.

1946b   "Organ Function and Form Perception." *Psychosomatic Medicine* 8/6, 367-385.

1948   "Psychodynamics in Parkinsonism." *Psychosomatic Medicine* 10/1, 1-14.

1949a   Conditions of Medical Responsibility." *The Review of Religion* 13, 241-258.

1949b   Review of Viktor von Weizsäcker, *Der Gestaltkreis* in *Psychosomatic Medicine* 11/2, 129-131.

1951   "Basic Concepts of Psychosomatic Medicine." *Pastoral Psychology,* January, 11-17. Reprinted in Simon Doniger (ed.), *Healing: Human and Divine,* 41-56. New York: Association Press, 1957. Citations from reprint in *Cross Currents* 7, 14-20, Winter, 1957.

1952a   Review of Ernst Kretschmer, *Medizinische Psychologie* in *Psychosomatic Medicine* 14, 510-511.

1952b   "The Meaning of Sex." *Pastoral Psychology* 3/26, 14-36. Reprinted in Simon Doniger (ed.), *Sex and Religion Today.* New York: Association Press, 1953.

1953a   "Hiltner a Moralist?" *Pastoral Psychology* 4/32, 59-60.

1953b   "Health from the Standpoint of the Physician." Paul B. Maves (ed.), *The Church and Mental Health,* 3/17. New York: Scribner's.

1953c   Review of F.S. Rothschild, *Das Ich und die Regulationen des Erlebnisvorgangs* in *Psychosomatic Medicine* 15, 363-365.

1954a   "Science and Spiritual Healing." *Pastoral Psychology* 5/44, 21-25. Citations from reprint in Simon Doniger (ed.), *Healing: Human and Divine,* 217-228. New York: Association Press, 1957.

1954b   Review of John W. Perry, *The Self in Psychotic Process: Its Symbolization in Schizophrenia* in *The Review of Religion* 19, 85-87.

1954c   "Masturbation." *Pastoral Psychology* 5/48, 13-19.

1954d   "Problems of Authority for Individual Christians: Its Use and Abuse." *The Journal of Pastoral Care* 8/4, 203-217.

1954e   "Les Dimensions Parapsychologiques en Medicine." *Revue Metapsychique,* September/December, 112-121.

1955a   Review of Erich Neumann, *The Origin and History of Consciousness* in *The Review of Religion* 20, 90-92.

1955b   "Prevention vs. Treatment." Simon Doniger (ed.), *The Minister's Consultation Clinic,* 132-135. Great Neck, New York: Channel Press.

1955c   "Parapsychological Dimensions in Medicine." *Proceedings of the First International Conference of Parapsychological Studies.* Parapsychology Foundation, 41-44.

1955d   "An Observation on Psi Function in Plants." *Proceedings of the First International Conference of Parapsychological Studies.* Parapsychology Foundation, 88-91.

1956a   "Telepathy: Discussion of Ehrenwald Paper." *The Psychiatric Quarterly* 30, 21-25 (reprint).

1956b   "Art and Rorschach." *Bennington College Alumnae Quarterly* 7/2, 3-12.

1956c   Review of C.G. Jung, *The Interpretation of Nature and the Psyche: Synchronicity, An Acausal Connecting Principle* in *The Review of Religion* 21, 84-87.

1957   "Rorschach Method in Unorthodox Healing." *Proceedings of Four Conferences of Parapsychological Studies*, 77-80.

1958a   Review of C.G. Jung, *Symbols of Transformation* in *The Review of Religion* 22, 203-207.

1958b   *The Psychological Examination of Candidates for the Ministry.* New York: Academy of Religion and Mental Health, 30 pp. Reprinted in Hans Hofmann (ed.), *The Ministry and Mental Health,* 101-126. New York: Association Press, 1960.

1959c   "Unconscious Motivation in the Choice of the Ministry as Vocation." *Pastoral Psychology* 9/89, 18-24. Reprinted in Wayne Oates (ed.), *The Minister's Own Mental Health.* Great Neck, NY: Channel Press, 1961.

1959d   Review of F.S. Rothschild, *Das Zentralnervensystem als Symbol Erlebens* in *Psychosomatic Medicine* 21, 77-80.

1960   "The Role of Physical Form in Psychodynamics." *Psychoanalysis and the Psychoanalytic Review* 47/1, 51-62.

1961   "On Masturbation." *Pastoral Psychology* 12/114, 53-56.

1962a   "Booth, Fromm, and Jung." *Pastoral Psychology* 13/124, 54-55.

1962b   "Healing the Sick." *Pastoral Psychology* 13/125, 11-24.

1962c   "Disease as a Message." *Journal of Religion and Health* 1/4, 309-318.

1963a   "Tests and Therapy Applied to the Clergy." *Journal of Religion and Health* 2/4, 267-276.

1963b   "Values in Nature and in Psychotherapy." *Archives of General Psychiatry* 8, 22-32.

1963c   "Biological Types and Forms of Religion." Unpublished address presented at the 23rd Annual Memorial Meeting of the Schilder Society, January 24, 1963.

1964a   "The Voice of the Body." Introduction to Aarne Siirala, *The Voice of Illness*, 1-25. Fortress. Citations from reprint in D. Belgum (ed.), *Religion and Medicine*, 96-117. Ames, IA: Iowa University Press, 1967.

1964b   "Cancer and Humanism (Psychosomatic Aspects of Evolution)." In (eds.) D.M. Kissen and L.L. LeShan, *Psychosomatic Aspects of Neoplastic Disease*, 159-169. London: Pitman Medical.

1964c   "Krebs und Tuberkulose im Rorschachschen Formdeutever-such." *Zeitschrift für Psychosomatische Medizin* 10, 176-188.

1965   "Irrational Complications of the Cancer Problem." *American Journal of Psychoanalysis* 25/1, 41-57.

1966   "The Cancer Patient and the Minister," *Pastoral Psychology* 17/161, 15-24.

1967a   "Physicians, Clergymen, and the Hospitalized Patient." *Journal of the American Medical Association* 200/4, 354-355.

1967b   "The Psychosomatic Object Relationship in Cancer." *Acta Medica Psychosomatica: Proceedings of the 7th European Conference on Psychosomatic Research*, 3-6 (reprint). Rome.

1969a   "The Auspicious Moment in Somatic Medicine." *The American Journal of Psychoanalysis* 29/1, 84-88.

1969b   "General and Organ-Specific Object Relationships in Cancer." *Annals of the New York Academy of Sciences* 164, 568-577.

1970a   Review of Ralph Weltge (ed.), *The Same Sex: An Appraisal of Homosexuality* in *Pastoral Psychology* 21/200, 55-59.

1970b   "Pastoral Psychology: The Next 20 Years in Ministry to the Sick." *Pastoral Psychology* 21/201, 22-27.

1972   "The Prevention and Cure of Cancer," Unpublished address for the National Federation of Spiritual Healers, April 29, 1972.

1973   "Psychobiological Aspects of 'Spontaneous' Regressions of Cancer." *Journal of American Academy of Psychoanalysis* 1/3, 303-317.

1974a   "The Biological Roots of the Generation Gap." *Psychiatria Fennica.* n.v., 111-118.

1974b   "Cancer and the Psyche." *International Mental Health Research Newsletter* 16/1, 15-16.

1974c   "Jung's and Rorschach's Contributions Toward a Psychobiological

Typology (An Example of Whitehead's Concept of Process)." *Toward a Discovery of the Person,* 68-73. Burbank, CA: Society for Personality Assessment.

1975   "Three Psychological Paths Toward Death: Cardiovascular Disease, Tuberculosis, and Cancer." *Bulletin of the New York Academy of Medicine* 51/3, 415-431.

1977   "A Spontaneous Recovery from Cancer." *Journal of the American Academy of Psychoanalysis.* 5/2, 207-214.

Works Cited in the Text

Abel, T. 1948. The Rorschach test in the study of cultures. *J. Projective Techniques.* 12:79.

Abel, T. 1954. *Themes in French Culture.* (eds.) R. Metraux and M. Mead Stanford Univ. Press.

Abelin, T. 1965. Cancer and smoking in Switzerland: Analysis of all patients who died of lung cancer in Switzerland 1951-1960. *Schw. Med. Wachr.* 95:233.

Abraham, K. 1925. *Psychoanalytische Studien zur Charakterbildung.* Vienna: Internat. Psychoanalytscher Verlag.

Abrams, R., and Finesinger, J.E. 1953. Guilt reactions in patients with cancer. *Cancer* 6:474.

Abrams, S. and Neubauer, P. 1975. Object orientedness: the person or the thing. *Psychiatric Quarterly.*

Adair, F.E. and Bagg, H.J. 1925. Breast stasis as the cause of mammary cancer. *Internat. Clin.* 4:19.

Am. Humane Assoc. Children's Division 1963. *Child Abuse.*

Anderson, M.R. 1964. Variations in the induction of chemical carcinogenesis. *Nature.* 204:35.

Andervont, H.B. 1944. Influence of environment on mammary cancer in mice. *J. Nat. Cancer Inst.* 4:579-581.

Antonelli, F. and Seccia, M. 1956. *Psiche e Tuberculosi.* Roma: Instituto di Medicina Sociale.

Ariel, T.M., and Pack, G.T. 1960. Cancer in infancy and childhood. *N. Y. J. Med.* 60:409.

Auster, L. 1965. Genital cancer in Jews. *N. Y. State J. Med.* 65:266.

Bacon, C.L., Renneker, R. and Cutler, M. 1952. A psychosomatic survey of cancer of the breast. *Psychosom. Med.* 14:453.

Bagg, H.J. 1936. Functional activity and mammary cancer in mice. *Amer. J. Cancer.* 27:542.

Balint, M. 1965. *Primary Love and Psychoanalytic Technique.* 2nd ed. New York: Liveright.

Balint, M. 1968. *The Basic Fault.* London: Tavistock.

Barnes, B.O. 1960. One factor in increase of bronchial carcinoma. *J.A.M.A.* 174:229.

Beecher, H.K. 1962. Nonspecific forces surrounding disease and the treatment of disease. *J.A.M.A.* 179:437.

Berkson, J. 1960. Smoking and cancer of the lungs. *Proc. Staff Meetings Mayo Clinic.* 35:367.

Berkson, J. 1962. Smoking and lung cancer: Another view. *Lancet* 1:807.

Berkson, J. 1963. Smoking and lung cancer. *Amer. Stat.* 17:15-22.

Bilz, R.. 1936. *Psychogene Angina.* Leipzig: S. Hirzel.

Blake, W. 1825. *Illustrations of the Book of Job.* New York, Morgan Library, 1935.

Boisen, A. 1935. *The Exploration of the Inner World.* Chicago: Clark Willett & Co.

Boisen, A. 1960. *Out of the Depths.* New York: Harper Brothers.

Borstelmann, L.J., Fowler, J.A., and McBryde, A. 1965. Maternal values, personalities and infant feeding. *Am. J. Orthopsychiatry* 35:302.

Bozeman, M.F., Orbach, C.E., and Sutherland, G.M. 1955. Psychological impact of cancer and its treatment. Part 1. *Cancer* 8:1.

Braden, C.S. 1954. A study of spiritual healing in the churches, *Pastoral Psychology.* 44:9.

Brenneman, J. 1942. *Practice of Pediatrics.* Hagerstown, Md.: Prior.

Breuning, H. 1908. *Geschichte der kuenstlichen Saeuglingsernaehrung.* Stuttgart: Enke.

Bruch, H. 1952. *Don't Be Afraid of Your Child.* New York: Farrar & Straus.

Buber, M. 1937. *I and Thou.* Edinburgh: Clark & Clark.

Campbell, J. 1959. *The Masks of God: Primitive Mythology.* New York: Viking.

Cherry, T. 1924, 1925. Cancer and acquired resistance to tuberculosis. *Med. J. Australia* 1:582 and 2:372.

Chichester, F. 1964. *The Lonely Sea and the Sky.* London: Hodder & Stoughton.

Christopherson, W.M. and Parker, J.E. 1965. Cervical cancer and its relation to early childbearing. *New Eng. J. Med.* 273: 235.

Clifton, E.E. and Irani, B. 1970. Pulmonary tuberculosis and cancer. *N. Y. State. J. of Med.* 70:274.

Cobb, B. 1962. Cancer. *Psychologic Practices with Physically Disabled.* (eds.) I. Garrett and E. Levine. New York: Columbia Univ. Press.

Collas, R. 1964. Psychosomatic considerations of the occurrence of cancer in male tuberculosis patients. *Psychosomatic Aspects of Neoplastic Disease.* (eds.) D.M. Kissen and L.L. LeShan. London: Pitman.

Coppen, A.J. and Metcalfe, M. 1964. Cancer and extraversion. *Psychosomatic Aspects of Neoplastic Disease.* (eds.) D.M. Kissen and L.L. LeShan. London: Pitman.

Crile, G. Jr. 1955. *Cancer and Common Sense.* New York: Viking.

Curtius, F. 1959. *Individuum and Krankheit.* Berlin.

Davis, C.M. 1928. Self-selection of diets by newly weaned infants. *Amer. J. Dis. Child.* 36:651 and *J.Amer. Dental Assoc.* 18:1142, 1931.

Dean, G. 1959. Lung cancer among white South Africans. *Brit. Med. J.* 31:853.

Dean, G. 1961. Lung cancer among white South Africans. Report on a further study. *Brit. Med. J.* 2:1599.

Dean, G. 1962. Lung cancer in Australia. *Med. J. Australia.* 49:1003.

DeLestapis. 1964. Sexuality and the modern world. *Cross Currents.* 14:162.

Dettweiler, P. 1877. Zur Physiotherapie der Gegenwart. *Berl. Klin. Wschr.* 14:511, 528, 560.

Doll, R. 1955. Etiology of Lung Cancer. *Advances Cancer Res.* 3:1.

Doll, R. 1965. Cancer the possibilities. *Brit. Med. J.* 1:471.

Doll, R. and Hill, A.B. 1952. A study of the aetiology of 'carcinoma of the lung. *Brit. Med. J.* 2:1271-1286.

Doll, R. and Hill, A.B. 1964. Mortality in relation to smoking. Ten years observations of British Doctors. *Brit. Med. J.* 1:1399-1410; concluded 1:1460-1467.

Doll, R. and Hill, A.B. 1966. Mortality of British doctors in relation to smoking: Observations on coronary thrombosis. *Epidemiological Approaches to the Study of Cancer and Other Diseases.* (ed.) W. Haenazel. *Nat. Can. Inst. Monog.* No. 19:205-268.

Drake, T.G.H. 1948. American infant feeding bottles. *J. Hist. Med.* 3:507.

Dubos, R. and Dubos, J. 1952. *The White Plague (Tuberculosis, Man and Society)*. Boston: Little, Brown & Co.

Dubos, R. 1959. *Mirage of Health.* New York: Harper.

Dubos, R. 1965. *Man Adapting.* New Haven: Yale Univ. Press.

Eastcott, D. 1956. The Epidemiology of Cancer in New Zealand. *Lancet* 270:37.

Ebstein, E. 1932. *Tuberkulose als Schicksal.* Stuttgart: Enke.

Ellenberger, H. 1954. Hermann Rorschach, M.D. *Bull. Menninger Clinic.* 18:173.

Ellenberger, H. 1958. Personal Communication.

Ellenberger, H. 1970. *The Discovery of the Unconscious: The History and Evolution of Dynamic Psychiatry.* New York: Basic Books.

Engel, G. 1954. Selection of clinical material in psychosomatic medicine: The need for a new physiology. *Psychosom. Med.* 16:368.

Erikson, E.H. 1963. *Childhood and Society.* 2nd ed. New York: W.W. Norton & Co.

Evans, E. 1926. *A Psychological Study of Cancer.* New York: Longmans, Green.

Everson, T.C. and Cole, W.H. 1966. *Spontaneous Regression of Cancer.* Philadelphia: W.B. Saunders.

Eysenck, H.J. 1965. *Smoking, Personality and Health.* New York: Basic Books.

Fiddian, J.V. 1930. The cell evolution theory of cancer. *Cambridge Univ. Med. Soc. Magazine.* 3:36.

Fisher, Sir R.A. 1959. *Smoking: The Cancer Controversy.* Edinburgh and London: Oliver & Boyd.

Flocks, R.H. 1965. Clinical cancer of the prostate. *J.A.M.A.* 193:89.

Forest, M.G., et al. 1973. Evidence of testicular activity in early infancy. *J. Clin. Endocrinol. Metabol.* 37:148.

Forgue, E. 1931. Le probleme du cancer dans ses aspects psychiques. *Gaz. des Hopitaux.* 104:827.

Franks, L.M. 1932. *Medical News.* June 2, 1961.

Franks, L.M. 1954. Latent carcinoma of the prostate. *J. Path. & Bact.* 68:603.

Franks, L.M. 1956. Latency and progression in tumors. *Lancet.* 2:1037.

Fras, I. and Litkin, E.M. 1966. Comparison of psychiatric symptoms in carcinoma of the pancreas and in two other intra-abdominal neoplasms. *Am. Psychiatr. Assoc. Meeting,* 1966.

French, L.M. and Alexander, F. 1941. *Psychogenic factors in bronchial asthma.* 2 vol. Washington: Psychosom. Med. Monographs.

French, L. and Alexander, F. 1964. *Psychoanalytic Therapy.* New York.

Freud, S. 1908. The most prevalent form of degradation in erotic life. *Coll. Papers.* 4:203.

Freud, S. 1909. Character and anal erotism. *Coll. Papers.* 2:45.

Freud, S. 1917. Mourning and melancholia. *Coll. Papers.* 4:152 London: Hogarth.

Freud, S. 1920. Beyond the pleasure principle. *Standard Edition,* vol. 18. London: Hogarth 1953.

Freud, S. 1930. *Civilization and Its Discontents.* New York: Doubleday, 1958.

Freud, S. 1937. Analysis terminable and interminable. *Coll. Papers.* 5:316.

Freud, S. 1962. On beginning the treatment. *The Complete Psychological Works of Sigmund Freud.* vol. 12. London: Hogarth, 1962.

Friedman, M. and Rosenman, R.H. 1974. *Type A Behavior and Your Heart.* New York: Knopf.

Fromm, E. 1947. *Man for Himself: An Inquiry into the Psychology of Ethics.* Greenwich, Conn: Fawcett.

Fullerton, D.T., Kollar, E.J. and Caldwell, A.B. 1962. A clinical study of ulcerative colitis. *J.A.M.A.* 181:463.

Gagnon, F. 1950. Contributions to the study of the etiology and prevention of cancer of the cervix of the uterus. *Am. J. Obsts. Gyn.*

Gengerelli, J.A. and Kiskner, F.J. 1954, eds. *The Psychological Variables of Cancer.* Berkeley & Los Angeles.

Gerami, S. and Cole, F.H. 1969. Coexisting carcinoma of the lung and pulmonary tuberculosis. *Ann. of Thoracic Surgery.* 7:317.

Geyl, P. 1965a. *The Netherlands in the Seventeenth Century.* 2nd vol. New York: Barnes & Noble.

Geyl, P. 1965b. *History of the Low Countries. Episodes and Problems.* London: MacMillan.

Goethe. 1825. *Goethe-Zelter Briefwechsel.* Leipzig, Reclam, 1902.

Gold, M.G. 1964. Causes of patients' delay in diseases of the breast. *Cancer.* 17:564-577.

Goldsen, R.K. Gerhard, R.P., and Handy, H.V. 1957. Some factors related to the patient delay in seeking diagnosis for cancer symptoms. *Cancer.* 10:1.

Greenberg, S.D. 1964. Coexistence of carcinoma and cancer of the lung. *Am. Rev. Resp. Dis.* 90:67.

Greenberg, D.S. 1975. A critical look at cancer coverage. *Columbia Journalism Review.* Jan/Feb. 1975:40.

Greene, W.A. 1958/59. Role of a vicarious object in the adaptation to object loss. *Psychosom. Med.* 20:344 & 21:438.

Greene, W.A. 1958/59. Role of a vicarioces object in the adaptation to object loss. *Psychosom. Med.* 20:344 & 21:438.

Grinker, R. et al. 1961. *The Phenomena of Depression.* New York: Paul B. Hoeber, Inc.

Groddeck, G., 1923. *The Book of the It.* London: Vision Press. 1969.

Gunther, I. 1949. *Death Be Not Proud.* London: Hamish Hamilton.

Hagstrum, J.H. 1964. *William Blake: Poet and Painter.* Chicago: Univ. of Chicago Press.

Hammond, E.C. and Horn, D. 1958. Smoking and death rates—report on 44 months of follow-up of 187,783 men. *J.A.M.A.* 166:1294.

Hare, E.H. 1962. Masturbating insanity. The history of an idea. *J. Men. Sci.* 108:1.

Harlow, H.F. and Harlow M.K. 1965. The affectional systems. *Behavior of Nonhuman Primates.* (eds.) G.M. Schrier, H.F. Harlow and F. Stolnitz. New York: Academic Press.

Harrison, T.R. 1966. The most distressing symptom. *J.A.M.A.* 198:170.

Haybittle, J.T. 1963. Mortality rates from cancer and tuberculosis. *Brit. J. Prev. Soc. Med.* 17:23-28.

Hayflick, L. 1966. Cell culture and aging phenomenon. *Topics in the Biology of Aging.* (ed.) P.K. Krohn. New York: Wiley.

Heinshiemer, H.W. 1968. *Best Regards to Aida.* New York: Knopf.

Helfer, R. and Kempe, C.H. 1968. *The Battered Child.* Chicago: Univ. of Chicago Press.

Hermann, I. 1936. Sich-Anklammaern Auf-Suche-Gehen. *Int. Z. Psycho-anal.* 22:349-370.

Hession, Brian. 1957. *Determined To Live.* New York: Doubleday.

Hinkle, L.E., et al. 1968. Occupation, education and coronary heart disease. *Science.* 161:238-46.

Hoernecke, G. and Berndt, H. 1965. Familial history of patients with cancer. *Schw. Med. Wachr.* 95:1161.

Hoyt, E.P. 1964. *A Gentleman of Broadway.* Boston: Little, Brown & Co.

Inman, W.S. 1961. Can a blow cause cancer? *Brit. J. Med. Psych.* 34:271.

Jaffe, J. and Slote, W.H. 1958. Interpersonal factors in denial of illness. *Arch. Neur. & Psychiatry.* 80:653.

John XXIII, Pope. 1965. *Diary of a Soul.* New York: McGraw-Hill.

Jones, E. 1953. *The Life and Work of Sigmund Freud.* 3 vol. New York: Basic Books.

J.A.M.A. 1934. Editorial: On Coley's Toxin. *J.A.M.A.* 103:1071.

Jung, C.G. 1923. *Psychological Types.* Trans. Pantheon, N.Y. 1958.

Kavetsky, R.E., Turkewich, N.M., and Balitsky, K.P. 1966. On the psychophysiological mechanism of the organism's resistance to tumor growth. *Ann. N.Y. Acad. Sci.* 125:933.

Keynes, J.M. 1936. *The General Theory of Employment, Interest and Money.* New York: Harcourt, Brace & Co.

Kinsey, A.C., Pomeroy, W.B., and Martin, C.E. 1948. *Sexual Behavior in the Human Male.* Phil: Saunders.

Kinsey, A.C. et al. 1953. *Sexual Behavior in the Human Female.* Phil: Saunders.

Kissen, D.M. 1958. Some psychosocial aspects of pulmonary tuberculosis. *Int. J. Social Psychiatry.* 3:252.

Kissen, D.M. 1960. Emotional factors in cigarette smoking and relapse in pulmonary tuberculosis. *Health Bul.* (Scotland) 18:38.

Kissen, D.M. 1963. Personality characteristics in males conducive to lung cancer. *Brit. J. Med. Psychol.* 36:27-36.

Kissen, D.M. 1964a. Lung cancer, inhalation, and personality. *Psychosomatic Aspects of Neoplastic Disease.* (eds.) D.M. Kissen and L.L. LeShan. London: Pitman.

Kissen, D.M. 1964b. Relationship between lung cancer, cigarette smoking, inhalation and personality. *Brit. J. Med. Psychol.* 37:203-216.

Kissen, D.M. 1965. Possible contribution of the psychosomatic approach to prevention in cancer. *Int. Psychosom. Cancer Study Group.* 4th Int. Conf. on Psychosom. Aspects of Neoplastic Disease. Turin, June 1965.

Kissen, D. 1966. The significance of personality in lung cancer in men. *Ann. N. Y. Head. Sci.* 125(3):820-826.

Korkes, L.L. and Lewis, N.D.C. 1955. An analysis of the relationship between psychological patterns and outcome of pulmonary tuberculosis. *J. Nerv. Ment. Dis.* 122:524.

Koroljow, S. 1962. Two cases of malignant tumors with metastases apparently treated successfully with hypoglycemic coma. *Psychiat. Quart.* 36:1-10.

Kowal, S.J. 1953. Emotions as a cause of cancer. *Psa. Review.* 42:217.

Kropotkin, P. 1902. *Mutual Aid, a Factor in Evolution.* New York: McClure, Phillips.

Kruse, H.D. 1964. The Golden Egg. *Bull. N. Y. Acad. Med.* 40:600.

LeShan, L.L. and Worthington, R.E. 1956. Some recurrent life history patterns observed in patients with malignant diseases. *J. Nerv. Ment. Dis.* 124:469.

LeShan, L.L. 1959. Cancer and personality: a critical review. *J. Nat. Cancer Inst.* 22:1-18.

LeShan, L.L. 1959. Psychological states as factors in the development of malignant disease. *J. Nat. Cancer Inst.* 22:1-18.

LeShan, L.L. and LeShan, E. 1961. Psychotherapy and the patient with a limited lifespan. *Psychiatry.* 24:318.

LeShan, L.L. 1965. Discussion following Booth's article in *American Journal of Psychoanalysis,* 1965.

LeShan, L.L. 1966. An emotional life history pattern associated with neoplastic disease. *Ann. N. Y. Acad. Sci.* 125:780-783.

Lewis, N.D.C. 1924. A discussion of the relationship of the chemical, physical and psychological aspects of personality. *Psa. Review.* 11:403.

Liddel, H.S. 1942. The alteration of the instinctual processes by conditioned reflexes. *Psychosom. Med.* 4:390.

Lorenz, K. 1966. *On Aggression.* New York: Harcourt, Brace and World.

MacDonald, I. 1942. Mammary carcinoma. Review of 2636 cases. *Surg. Jour. Gyn. Obst.* 74:75.

McGovern, G.P., Miller, D.H., and Robertson, E.E. 1959. A mental syndrome associated with lung carcinoma. *Arch. Neur. Psychiatry.* 81:341.

McKegney, F., Isay, R.A., and Balsam, A. 1965. The problem of the dying patient. *N. Y. J. Med.* 65:2356.

McLuhan. 1964. *Understanding Media: The Extensions of Man.* New York: McGraw-Hill.

Malcolm, N. 1958. *Ludwig Wittgenstein, A Memoir.* Oxford: Oxford Paperbacks.

Marcial, V.G. 1960. Socioeconomic aspects of the incidence of cancer in Puerto Rico. *Culture, Society and Health.* (ed.) V. Rubin; *N. Y. Acad. Sci.* 84:981.

Masserman, J.H. and Siever, P. 1944. Dominance, neurosis and aggression. *Psychosom. Med.* 6:7-16.

Masters, W.H. and Johnson, V.E. 1970. *The Pleasure Bond.* Boston, Toronto: Little, Brown & Co.

Mead, M. 1964. *Continuities in Cultural Evolution.* New Haven and London: Yale Univ. Press.

Meerloo, J.A.M. 1944. The initial neurologic and psychiatric syndrome of pulmonary growth. *J.A.M.A.* 126:558.

Meerloo, J.A.M. 1954. Psychological implications of malignant growth. *Brit. J. Med. Psychol.* 27:210.

Merei, F. 1953. *Der Aufforderungscharakter der Rorschach Tafeln.* Ivonsbruck: Institut für Psychodiagnostik und angewandte Psychologie.

Minkowska, F. 1956. *Le Rorschach.* Brussells: Brouwer.

Mitchell, J.S. 1960. *Studies in Radiotherapeutics.* Oxford: Blackwell.

Mittleman, N., Wolff, H.G. and Scharf, M. 1942. Experimental studies on patients with gastritis, duodenitis and peptic ulcer. *Psychosom. Med.* 4:4.

National Society for the Prevention of Cruelty to Children. *Ann. Reports* 1959-1966. London WI, 1-3 Riding House Str.

Nauts, H.C., Fowler, G.A., and Bogatko, F.H. 1953. *A Review of the Influence of Bacterial Infection and Bacterial Products (Coleys' Toxins) on Malignant Tumors in Man.* Stockholm.

Newton, N. and Newton, M. 1967. Psychological aspects of lactation. *New Eng. J. Med.* 277:1179.

Orbach, C.E., Sutherland, A.M., and Bozeman, A.F. 1955. Psychological impact of cancer and its treatment. Part 2. *Cancer.* 8:20.

Paget, J. 1870. *Surgical Pathology.* 2nd ed. London: Longmans, Green.

Parker, W. 1885. *Cancer: A Study of Ninety-Seven Cases of Cancer of the Female Breast.* New York.

Passey, R.D. 1962. Some problems in lung cancer. *Lancet.* 2:107.

Pendergrass, E.P. 1961. Host resistance and other intangibles in the treatment of cancer. *Roentg. Radium Ther., Nucl. Med.* 85:891.

Pereyra, A.J. 1961. Cervical cancer and sex activity. *Obst. & Gyn.* 17:154.

Perrin, G.M. and Pierce, I.R. 1959. Psychosomatic aspects of cancer: A review. *Psychosom. Med.* 21:397.

Perrott, G. St. J. 1945. The problem of chronic disease. *Psychosom. Med.* 7:21.

Peyser, Joan. 1975. Section on Historical Medicine. *N. Y. Academy of Med.* April 23, 1975.

Philipe, A. 1963. *Le Temps d'un Soupir.* Paris: Jouillard.

Phillips, L. and Smith, G.S. 1953. *Rorschach Interpretation.* New York.

Piel, G. 1964. Physician, heal thy society. *Bull. N. Y. Acad. Med.* 40:615.

Pike, M.C. and Doll, R. 1965. Age at onset of lung cancer: Significance in relation to effect of smoking. *Lancet.* 1:665.

Piotrowski, Z. 1957. *Perceptanalysis.* New York: Macmillan Co.

Planck, M. 1949. *Scientific Autobiography and Other Papers.* New York: Greenwood Press, 1968. p 34.

Portmann, A. 1956. *Biologie und Geist.* Zurich: Rhin Verlag.

Portmann, A. 1962. *New Pathways in Biology.* New York: Harper & Row.

Prichard, J.S., Schwab, R. and Tillmann, W. 1951. The effects of stress and the results of medication in different personalities with Parkinson's disease. *Psychosom. Med.* 13:106.

Purcell, K. 1965. Critical appraisal of psychosomatic studies of asthma. *N.Y. State J. Med.* 25:106.

Quisenberry, W.B. 1960. Sociological factors in cancer in Hawaii. *Culture, Society and Health.* (ed.) V. Rubin. *N.Y. Acad. Sci.* 84:795.

Rabinowitch, E. 1964. James Franck and Leo Szilard. *Bull. of Atomic Scientists.* Oct. 1964:16.

Rassidakis, N.C. 1974. Schizophrenia, psychosomatic illnesses, diabetes mellitus and malignant neoplasms. *Int. Ment. Health Res. News.* 16:1.

Reagan, M.D. 1964. For a guaranteed income. *New York Times Mag.* 7 June 1964.

Renneker, R.E., Cutler, R., and Hora, J. 1963. Psychoanalytical exploration of emotional correlates of cancer of the breast. *Psychosom. Med.* 25:106.

Richter, C.P. 1941. Biology of drives. *Psychosom. Med.* 3:105-110.

Richter, C.P. 1959. The phenomenon of sudden unexplained death in animals and men. in *The Meaning of Death.* (ed.) H. Fiefel, New York: Blakiston Co.

Ritey, H. Personal Communication.

Robbins, J. and Robbins, I. 1954. The great untold story of Senator Taft: Eight weeks to live. *This Week.* Jan. 17, 1954:8.

Roemer, G.C. 1937. Vom Rorschach Test zum Symboltest. *Zentralblatt Psychotherapie.* 10:310.

Rorschach, H. 1921. *Psychodiagnostik.* Bern: E. Birscher.

Rosenblith, W.A. Social consequences of change. Proc. Am. Acad. Arts & Sci. *Daedalus.* Summer 1961:512.

Rotkin, I.D. 1962. Relation of adolescent coitus to cervical cancer risk. *J.A.M.A.* 179:486.

Rotkin, I.D., Quenk, N., and Couchman, M. 1965. Psychosexual factors and cervical cancer. *Arch. Gen. Psychiatry.* 13:532.

Ruhräh, J. 1925. *Pediatrics of the Past.* New York: Hoeber.

Rusk, H. 1966. The battered child. *New York Times.* Mar. 27. p. 83.

Sacerdote, P. 1964. Pain relief through hypnotherapy. *Psychosomatic Aspects of Neoplastic Disease.* (eds.) D.M. Kissen & L.L. LeShan. London: Pitman.

Salk, J. 1969. Immunological paradoxes: Theoretical considerations in the rejection or retention of grafts, tumors, and normal tissue. *Ann. N.Y. Acad. Sci.* 164:365-379.

Salk, J. 1971. Personal Communication.

Schloesser, P. 1964. The abused child. *Bull. Menninger Clinic* 28:260.

Schumer, W.R. and Sperling, R. 1968. Shock and its effect on the cell. *J.A.M.A.* 205:215.

Schwartz, P. 1960. Pulmonary cancer and pulmonary tuberculosis. *Act. Tuberc. Scand.* 38:195.

Searles, H.F. 1960. *The Nonhuman Environment.* New York: Int. Univ. Press.

Seay, B., Alexander, B.K., and Harlow, H.F. 1964. Maternal behavior of socially deprived rhesus monkeys. *J. Abn. Soc. Psych.* 69:345.

Sechehaye, M.A. 1951. *Symbolic Realization.* New York: Int. Univ. Press.

Seltzer, C.C. 1963. Morphologic constitution and smoking. *J.A.M.A.* 183:639.

Selye, H. 1967. *In Vivo (The Case for Supramolecular Biology).* New York: Liverwright.

Schroedinger, E. 1945. *What Is Life?* New York: Macmillan.

Schur, M. 1972. *Freud Living and Dying.* New York: Int. Univ. Press.

Shapiro, A.K. 1963. Psychological aspects of medication in *The Psychological Basis of Medical Practice.* H.I. Lief, V.F. Lief and N.R. Lief. New York: Hoeber.

Sherrington, Sir C. 1941. *Man on His Nature.* New York: Macmillan.

Shrifte, M. 1962. Toward identification of a psychological variable in host resistance to cancer. *Psychosom. Med.* 24:390.

Sigergist, H.E. 1932. The historical development of the pathology and therapy of cancer. *Bull. N.Y. Acad. Med.* 8:642.

Smithers, D.W. 1964. *On the Nature of Neoplasia in Man.* Edinburgh: Livingstone.

Solzhenitsyn, A.I. 1968. *The Cancer Ward.* New York: Dial Press.

Spitz, R. 1945. Hospitalism: An inquiry into psychiatric conditions in early childhood. *The Psychoanalytic Study of the Child.* vol. 1. p. 53. New York: Int. Univ. Press.

Spitz, R. 1952. Authority and masturbation: Some remarks on a bibliographic investigation. *Psychoanal. Quart.,* 21.

Spitz, R. 1957. *No and Yes.* New York: Int. Univ. Press.

Spitz, R. 1965. *The First Year of Life.* New York: Int. Univ. Press.

Stehlin, J.S. and Beach, K.H. 1966. Psychological aspects of cancer therapy. *J.A.M.A.* 197:140.

Stengel, E. 1962. Recent research into suicide and attempted suicide. *A.J. Psychiatry.* 118:725.

Stephenson, H. and Grace, W.J. 1954. Life stress and cancer of the cervix. *Psychosom. Med.* 16:287.

Stevenson, D.L. 1964. Evolution and the neurobiogenesis of neoplasia. *Psychosomatic Aspects of Neoplastic Disease.* (eds.) D.M. Kissen and L.L. LeShan, London: Pitman.

Stone, L. 1965. Pieter Geyl. *The New York Review.* 8 April 1965, p. 29.

Sunley, R. 1958. Early American literature on child rearing. *Childhood in Contemporary Cultures.* (eds) M. Mead and M. Wolfenstein. Univ. of Chicago Press.

Sutherland, A.M. 1957a. The psychological impact of post-operative cancer. *Bull. N. Y. Acad. Med.* 32:428.

Sutherland, A.M. 1957b. Should the patients be told the truth about serious illness? Practitioners Conference. *N. Y. Medicine.* Jan. 5, p. 36.

Szondi, L. 1944. *Schickalsanalyse.* Basel: Schwabe.

Szondi. L. 1948. *Schicksalsanalyse.* 2nd ed. Basel: Schwabe.

Szondi, L., Moser, V., and Webb, M. 1959. *The Szondi Test.* Phila: Lippincott.

Tarlau, M. and Smalheiser, I. 1951. Personality patterns in patients with malignant tumors of the breast and cervix. *Psychosom. Med.* 13:117.

Theobald, R. 1965. *The Guaranteed Income.* New York: Doubleday.

Thomas, L. 1974. *The Lives of a Cell.* New York: Viking Press.

Thompson, E.P. 1964. *The Making of the British Working Class.* New York: Pantheon.

Time, 1957. Death of a surgeon. *Time Magazine.* March 18, p. 42 (p. 36 Can. ed.).

Time, 1965. No more triumphs? *Time Magazine.* April 23, p. 68 (p. 62 Can. ed.).

Tinbergen, N. 1955. *The Study of Instinct.* Oxford: Clarendon.

Tinbergen, E. and Tinbergen, N. 1973. Early childhood autism: An ethological approach. *Zeitschrift für Tierpsychologie.* Bieheft 10, 1973.

Titchener, J. and Levine, M. 1960. *Surgery as a Human Experience.* New York: Oxford.

Todd, G.F. 1959. *Statistics of Smoking.* Research Paper I, 2nd ed. Tobacco Research Council.

Tokuhata, G. and Lilienfeld, A.M. 1963. Familial aggregation of lung cancer in humans. *J. Nat. Cancer Inst.* 30:289.

Tosquelles, 1945. Le fascination au cours du Rorschach. *Rorschachiana* 1:108. Bern: Huber.

Towne, J.E. 1955. Carcinoma of the cervix in multiparous and celibate women. *Am. J. Obst. Gynec.* 69:616.

U.S. Public Health Service. 1964. *Surgeon General's Report on Smoking and Health.* Washington, D.C.

U.S. Public Health Service. 1974. *Cancer Rates and Risks,* 2nd ed.

U.S. Public Health Service. *Vital Statistics.* Washington, D.C. 1931, 1941, 1951, 1961, 1962.

Von Mueller, F. 1920. *J. Von Mering's Lehrbuch der inneren Medizin.* Jena: Fisher.

Von Uexkuell, J. 1921. *Umwelt und Innenwelt der Tiere.* 2nd ed. Berlin: Springer.

Von Weizsäcker, V. 1934. *Wege psychophysischer Forschung.* S. Ber. Heidelbg: Akad. Wiss. 1934, 4.

Von Weizsäcker, V. 1950. *Der Gestaltkreis.* 4th ed. Stuttgart: Thieme.

Warburg, O. 1926. *Ueber der Stoffwechsel der Tumoren.* Berlin.

Warburg, O. 1956. On the origin of cancer cells. *Science.* 123:309-314.

Warburg, O. 1964. Prefatory chapter. *Ann. Rev. Biochem.* 33:1-13.

Warburg, O. 1967. *The Prime Cause and Prevention of Cancer.* Eng. ed. Dean Burk 2nd rev. ed. 1969. Warzburg: K. Triltsh.

Warthin, A.S. 1913. Heredity with reference to carcinoma. *Arch. Int. Med.* 12:546-555.

Weinstock, C. 1974. Psychosocial rehabilitation of cancer patients: A pilot study. *Int. Ment. Health Res. News.* Fall, 1974: 10-14.

Weiss, D.W. 1969. Immunological parameters of the host-parasite relationship in neoplasia. *Ann. N.Y. Acad. Sci.* 164:431-438.

Westergren, A. 1959. One hundred cases of pulmonary carcinoma analysed with reference to tuberculosis. *Acta Chirug. Scand.* supp. 245, p. 121.

Wheeler, J.J. and Caldwell, B.M. 1955. Psychological evaluation of women with cancer of the breast and of the cervix. *Psychosom. Med.* 17:256.

Winnicott, D.W. 1953. Transitional objects and transactional phenomena: A study of the first not-me possession. *Int. J. Psa.* 34:89.

Wittkower, E. 1949. *A Psychiatrist Looks at Tuberculosis.* London: Nat. Assoc. Prev. Tuberc.

Whitehead, A.N. 1920. *The Concept of Nature.* Ann Arbor: Univ. of Michigan Press, 1957.

Whitehead, A.N. 1938. *Modes of Thought.* Cambridge: Cambridge Univ. Press, 1956.

Wolters, L. 1959. Arthur Godfrey's fight against cancer. *Today's Health.*

World Health Organization, 1965. Mortality from malignant neoplasm of larynx and of trachea, bronchus and lung 1950-1963. *Epidem. Vital Stat. Rep.* 18:316.